The Mindful Way

Managing Cancer Symptoms

DR CHERYL REZEK

sheldon PRESS

First published in Great Britain in 2019 by Sheldon Press, an imprint of John Murray Press. An Hachette UK company

1

Copyright © Dr Cheryl Rezek 2019

A CIP catalogue record for this title is available from the British Library

Paperback ISBN 978 1 847 09423 0

eBook ISBN 978 1 847 09424 7

Typeset by Cenveo® Publisher Services.

Printed and bound in Great Britain by Clays Ltd, Elcograf S.p.A.

John Murray policy is to use papers that are natural, renewable and recyclable products and made from wood grown in sustainable forests. The logging and manufacturing processes are expected to conform to the environmental regulations of the country of origin.

Sheldon Press
Carmelite House
50 Victoria Embankment
London EC4Y 0DZ

www.sheldonpress.co.uk

Thank you to Sophie Brown and Tom Davey

Contents

An important note about the text

To access the audio downloads that accompany this book, go to: www.lifehappens-mindfulness.com/book-audio

Do not listen to the audio material while driving or operating any machinery or item.

Disclaimer: This book makes no claim to act as a cure or treatment of any conditions, nor does it advocate discontinuation of any intervention or treatment.

1

Life happens

Life brings with it experiences and events that are sometimes wonderful and at other times distressing and difficult. Having cancer can leave you feeling vulnerable and despairing, filled with fear and frustration and perhaps terrified of the outcome. Life changes, it moves and shifts, it comes and goes. That is the very nature of life. It has little to do with whether we are good, caring, moral people or devious, mean and shameless. There is no fairness in life and having an illness has no reason or judgement behind it.

There are plenty of books and advice out there but no fool-proof manual on how to face and negotiate this shake up of your world. This book is not one either – it's highly unlikely that one exists as we're all different and what works for one person may be of little value to another. In this book, what is offered is not a cure or a false promise, not a manual that fills you with hope and then doesn't care about the outcome or the fallout. What it gives is an outline of an approach to life and what might assist you in navigating the good and the horrible.

At its foundation is a combination of psychological concepts gleaned from decades of clinical work interwoven with mindfulness and meditation as a way of managing life and all that it can bring. It doesn't hope to remove the cancer or all of your fears; it doesn't make any claims to transform your illness or your life; but what it does offer are ideas and concepts, mindfulness meditation practices and thoughts that look to soften the intense glare of your illness and to hold your hand as you walk down this road.

Mindfulness helps by building a strong and powerful anchor within you that you can call upon when dealing with difficult experiences. Life is complex and facing an illness that may require ongoing interventions and procedures, that may leave you physically and emotionally changed in some way, and that may or may not return, can involve a relentless barrage of different emotions and demands. It is not only terrifying, but it can also feel overwhelming and lead you to believe that you are powerless over it no matter what you do.

Switch on, not off

Mindfulness is about switching on, not switching off. Instead of zoning out, mindfulness meditation brings your awareness to your life right now, grounding you and allowing you to be alive in this moment. This makes it different from relaxation as your *intention* is to bring your *attention* to each moment as it unfolds, even when some of those moments are distressing or confusing.

The idea of 'intention'

You will often come across the concept of 'intention' in books on mindfulness. In short, it is about approaching whatever practice or action you are planning on undertaking with a specific purpose or intent. What is your aim when doing a practice? This helps to focus your mind and your energy when doing it. The aim may be to anchor yourself, to ease the physical tension in your body, to reconnect to the kindness or uncritical part of yourself, or something else.

There are meditations that specifically move you towards negotiating the cancer within you, such as meditating on the destructive cells being removed with each outbreath or imagining that your breath is a shower of health. These involve a greater degree of visualization and may be helpful to you. The concern is that should the cancer remain, return or spread, you may feel angry or disillusioned with meditation. It is for this reason that such meditations or visualizations are not included in this book as the meditations and practices provided throughout are non-specific and can be done no matter what your situation.

One of the useful things about mindfulness is that you can learn to step away from yourself. Developing this ability, through doing the practices, opens you to the possibility of using those split-second moments between thoughts, actions or emotions to choose what you want to do. Do I choose to go down this path or that one? Do I wish to impulsively react or to respond in a way that I would like to? There are many moments in our day where we have choice: a choice to self-criticize or a choice to accept; a choice to sink or a choice to use humour to cope. This links to the idea of intention. It's about having an intention about which choice or choices you want to make in this moment, and in those other moments of your life.

With practice and ongoing application (sadly, there is no quick fix or magic), developing this approach will offer you an alternative solution to how you perceive and react not only to your illness itself but to other aspects around it too, such as making difficult decisions, finding quiet within yourself, compassion, self-care and much more. This combined approach of psychology and mindfulness gives you a broad and inclusive framework in which to manage your perspective on life and how you navigate your illness. Another advantage of using it in your everyday life is that it increases your capacity to enjoy and appreciate other experiences, even while you are ill.

The foundation of the book

This book offers a gentle introduction to the model and how it can become an ally in coping with your cancer. It will cover some general information and statistics on cancer and how mindfulness has been proven to help with the symptoms of cancer. More importantly, it will guide you through each idea and mindfulness practice and give you the tools to help ease your suffering and fear, your distress and confusion. It will discuss sleep, pain management and how exercise before, during and after cancer is so beneficial, as well as provide a gentle series of movements and a walking meditation.

The truth is that no approach is going to transform your body back to the time when you were healthy or take your life and mind back to the pre-cancer phase. You can't go back no matter how hard you try, nor can you project yourself into the future and be certain of an outcome. What you can do, and what this book will emphasize repeatedly, is be here, right now, and live your life with truth and knowledge that you are doing so. That is your only certainty and it is within your control, so what are you going to do with it? Are you willing to renegotiate your relationship with your life?

Cancer will turn your life upside down and inside out. You may have no interest in reading any further. Your mind may be so overwhelmed by your illness, the procedures, the side effects, the fears and terrors and that dreaded uncertainty that there is no space in your head, or willingness in your heart, to think this book may have anything of use in it. That's fair enough and there may be nothing of interest here for you. However, if and when there might be a tiny space, read on and take from it whatever you wish. The book is an offering not a prescription.

Mindfulness practices and audio access to guided meditations

Throughout the book, mindfulness practices are outlined, and you are provided with step-by-step guidance on how to do them.

The audio of the guided practices is included as a MP3 download at www.lifehappens-mindfulness.com/book-audio.

When you see the symbol 🔊 it indicates that there is a guided practice that can be listened to from the audio download.

It is strongly recommended that you attempt all the practices, the written as well as those on the audio download, at least once. It cannot be emphasized enough how essential and important it is that you do the practices from the audio download. Over time, you will become more aware of which practices work best for you and it is highly likely you will feel some benefit from at least one of them.

Keep in mind that doing any of these practices once will change very little. Engaging with them consistently is the key factor in how effective mindfulness will be for managing your cancer experience and in life generally. The more you do the practices, the more engrained and useful mindfulness will become in your daily life – and the greater the benefits.

2

Cancer facts, figures and statistics

There are numerous types of cancer so rather than list them it is more appropriate to provide some information on cancer in general. The following will provide an overview of incidence worldwide, contributing factors, treatment types and side effects, and survival rates.

Cancer isn't an entity that has a mind or an ability to discriminate: it is a disease that can develop in anyone, regardless of age, gender, race or even lifestyle, diet or exercise regime. Factors may, or in some cases may not, contribute to it occurring but what is important is recognizing that some factors, such as smoking or alcohol consumption, do increase risk and that if you already have a diagnosis of cancer then it's even more important to take on board the necessity of balancing mind and body, whether it be through revisiting your approach to exercise and diet or your levels of stress.

General cancer statistics – UK and global

Cancer Research UK record the following figures for incidence of cancer in the UK:[1]

- There were 163,444 deaths from cancer in 2016.
- There were 359,960 new cases of cancer in 2015.
- In 2015, 38 per cent of cancer cases were preventable.
- One in two people born after 1960 will be diagnosed with some form of cancer in their lifetime.

- Smoking is the largest cause of cancer. Around a fifth of all cancer deaths are from lung cancer.
- In 2015, 52 per cent of new cases of cancer in males were prostate, lung or bowel cancer.
- In 2015, 54 per cent of new cases of cancer in females were breast, lung or bowel cancer.
- Breast cancer is the most common cancer, accounting for almost a sixth (15 per cent) of all cases in males and females combined in 2015. The next most common cancers are prostate (13 per cent), lung (13 per cent), and bowel (12 per cent). Although there are more than 200 types of cancer, just these four types – breast, prostate, lung and bowel – accounted for 53 per cent of all new cases in 2015.
- Cancer was the cause of 28 per cent of all deaths in 2016.
- Every four minutes someone in the UK dies from cancer.
- Each year 53 per cent of all cancer deaths are people aged 75 and over.
- 50 per cent of people diagnosed with cancer in England and Wales survive for ten years or more.
- Cancer survival is higher in women than men.
- Cancer survival is improving and has doubled over the last 40 years.
- Cancer survival is generally higher in people diagnosed at the age of 40 or younger, with the exception of breast, bowel and prostate cancer, where survival is highest in middle age.

The World Health Organization note the following statistics with regard to incidence of cancer worldwide:[2]

- 8.8 million people died from cancer worldwide in 2015. That is nearly one in six of all deaths.
- The estimated global total annual economic cost of cancer each year is US$1.16 trillion.

- Between 30 and 50 per cent of cancers could be prevented.
- Around one-third of deaths from cancer are due to the five leading behavioural and dietary risks: high body mass index, low fruit and vegetable intake, lack of physical activity, tobacco use and alcohol use.
- Approximately 70 per cent of deaths from cancer occur in low- and middle-income countries.
- Tobacco use is the most important risk factor for cancer and is responsible for approximately 22 per cent of cancer deaths.
- Cancer-causing infections, such as hepatitis and human papilloma virus (HPV), are responsible for up to 25 per cent of cancer cases in low- and middle-income countries.

Cancer Research UK provide further figures for worldwide rates of cancer:[3]

- It is estimated that worldwide there were 32.5 million men and women still alive in 2012 up to five years after their diagnosis. Most of these had been diagnosed with breast (females only), bowel (including anus) or prostate cancer.
- In 2012, an estimated 14.1 million new cases of cancer occurred worldwide.
- An estimated 169.3 million years of healthy life were lost globally because of cancer in 2008.
- Worldwide there will be 23.6 million new cases of cancer each year by 2030 (estimated).

Cancer Research UK also provide statistics relating to cancer in young people specifically:[4]

- There are around 2,600 new cancer cases in young people in the UK every year – more than seven every day.
- Among young people in the UK, cancer incidence rates are highest in those aged 20–24.

- Since the early 1990s, cancer incidence rates in young people have increased by 28 per cent in the UK. The increase is larger in females where rates have increased by almost 38 per cent than in males where rates have increased by 19 per cent.
- Over the last decade, cancer incidence rates in young people have increased by 11 per cent in the UK, although this includes an increase in females (20 per cent) and stable rates in males.
- Lymphomas, carcinomas and germ cell tumours account for almost a third of all cancers diagnosed in young people, with lymphomas the most common.

Statistics are also available for cancer in children:[5]

- There are around 1,800 new cancer cases in children in the UK every year – around five every day.
- Among children in the UK, cancer incidence rates are highest in those aged under four years old.
- From the early 1990s, incidence rates for cancers in children increased by 13 per cent in the UK, with rates in boys increasing by 11 per cent and rates in girls increasing by 15 per cent. However, over the last decade, incidence rates for cancers in children have remained stable in the UK.
- Leukaemia, brain, other central nervous system (CNS) and intracranial tumours and lymphomas account for more than two-thirds of all cancers diagnosed in children, with leukaemia the most common.
- It is estimated that around one child in 500 in the UK will be diagnosed with cancer by the age of 14.

Main contributing factors

The main contributing factors to cancer have been identified as the following:[6]

Smoking

Smoking accounts for more than one in four cancer deaths, and three in 20 cancer cases. Tobacco smoke contains many different chemicals that damage the DNA of your cells. Chemicals in the smoke enter the blood stream and affect the entire body. It can cause at least 15 types of cancer, including lung, nose, mouth, liver, stomach, kidney and pancreas. It usually takes many years for DNA damage from smoking to cause cancer, but research shows that for every 15 cigarettes smoked there is a DNA change which could cause a cell to become cancerous. Smoking causes seven in ten lung cancer cases in the UK.

Obesity and weight

Obesity is the UK's biggest cause of cancer after smoking. Extra fat does not just sit there – it sends signals which tell cells to divide more often which can cause cancer. Each year 22,800 cases of cancer in the UK could be prevented by maintaining a healthy weight. Consistent results from decades of research involving millions of people show the link between obesity and cancer. The risk increases as more weight is gained.

Sun and ultraviolet (UV) light

Overexposure to UV light from the sun or sunbeds is the main cause of skin cancer. We all need some vitamin D in order to have healthy bones, but we should be able to get enough without getting sunburnt. Applying after-sun lotion can soothe the skin, but it cannot repair any DNA damage. When the skin burns, genetic material is damaged in skin cells and can cause them to start growing out of control, which can lead to skin cancer.

Diet

A healthy diet can prevent around one in 20 cancers. A diet with plenty of fibre, fruit and vegetables, while eating less red meat, processed meat and salt can cut the risk. An unhealthy diet could increase the risk of mouth, throat, lung, stomach and bowel cancer. Fruit and vegetables provide healthy vitamins and minerals and help you maintain a healthy body weight.

Physical activity

Being active and maintaining a healthy weight reduces the risk of 13 types of cancer. Brisk walking, cycling and even housework can count towards activity. Activity can promote a healthy level of hormones in the body and assist with digestion and inflammation in the bowel.

Alcohol

Alcohol causes several types of cancer including breast, mouth and bowel. All types of alcohol increase cancer risk and it is one of the most well-researched causes. It is estimated to cause 3 per cent of cases each year. When you drink alcohol, cancer-causing chemicals are formed and hormone levels are affected.

Infections

Most people will be exposed to human papillomavirus (HPV) in their lifetime. Virtually all cervical cancer cases are caused by HPV, but it can also cause cancers in other areas like the vagina, vulva, penis, anus, mouth and throat. HPV causes cells to divide more than usual.

Only one in 1,000 cases of UK cancer are caused by HIV. Non-Hodgkin lymphoma and virtually all cases of Kaposi sarcoma are caused by HIV. Chronic infection with hepatitis B and hepatitis C can increase liver cancer and non-Hodgkin lymphoma risk. Epstein-Barr virus (EBV) is a very common infection that can increase the risk of some types of cancer including Hodgkin lymphoma.

Air pollution

Almost one in ten lung cancer cases in the UK are caused by exposure to outdoor air pollution. Exposure to second-hand smoke increases the risk of cancer as well as other diseases such as heart disease and stroke. Scientists have found that exposure to radon gas accounts for only 4 per cent of all UK cases of lung cancer.

Hormones

Hormone replacement therapy (HRT) can cause some types of cancer (breast, womb and ovarian), but this is small in comparison with other risk factors such as smoking or obesity. With regards to the contraceptive pill, the longer a woman takes it the higher her risk of cervical cancer is – nearly double the risk when taking it for more than five years. About 1 per cent of breast cancers are caused by oral contraceptives, however, the combined pill can protect against certain cancers such as ovarian and womb cancers, and the effects are bigger the longer it is taken.

Workplace causes

Scientists estimate that exposure to health hazards at work causes 4 per cent of cancer cases in the UK. Certain types of work carry higher risks.

- Agriculture, forestry and fishing – too much sun or exposure to agricultural chemicals
- Construction and painting – exposure to asbestos, too much sun, silica, diesel fumes, coal, paint and solvents or wood dust
- Manufacturing and mining – exposure to fossil fuels, asbestos, silica, solvents or too much sun
- Service industries – too much sun, second-hand smoke or engine fumes

Genes

Cancers due to inherited faulty genes are much less common than cancers caused by gene changes from aging or other factors. Genetic specialists estimate that between three and ten in every 100 cancers are linked to an inherited faulty gene.

Age

For every 100 people diagnosed with cancer, 89 will be aged over 50, 10 will be between 25 and 49 years old and one will be 24 years or under. This is because our cells get damaged over time, and the damage build-up can sometimes lead to cancer. Nine in ten cancer cases in the UK are people aged 50 and over.

Cancer controversies

There are some factors reported to contribute to cancer that are still controversial or lack scientific evidence to support the claim that they are harmful.

- Cosmetics and toiletries – there is no good scientific evidence to support a link between cosmetics and cancer.
- Mobile phones and Wi-Fi – non-ionizing radiation is produced but is not powerful enough to damage DNA.
- Plastic bottles – there is no evidence to back up claims that drinking fluids that have been stored in plastic bottles causes cancer.
- Stress – no direct link has been found but being stressed could lead to unhealthy lifestyle choices such as smoking or overeating which can increase the risk.

Treatment types and their side effects

There are several different types of treatment for cancer. Unfortunately, some do have side effects that may be temporary or permanent. Some people choose not to have treatment or to cease treatment after a certain period. That is a personal choice made because they prefer to live whatever time they have left in a specific way. For others, refusing treatment is not an option they would ever consider. It really is a very personal decision.

Surgery

Surgery when used to treat cancer is a procedure in which a surgeon removes cancer from your body. Surgery works best for solid tumours that are contained in one area. It is a local treatment, meaning that it treats only the part of your body with the cancer. It is not used for leukaemia (a type of blood cancer) or for cancers that have spread.

Risks include pain, infection, bleeding, damage to nearby tissues and a reaction to anaesthesia.

Radiation therapy

Radiation therapy (also called radiotherapy) is a cancer treatment that uses high doses of radiation to kill cancer cells and shrink tumours.

Drawbacks include the fact that there is a limit to how much radiation an area of your body can safely receive over the course of your lifetime, and that it can affect nearby healthy cells, causing damage and symptoms such as fatigue, hair loss, diarrhoea, vomiting, headaches, skin changes and swelling.

Chemotherapy

Chemotherapy is a type of cancer treatment that uses drugs to kill cancer cells. It works by stopping or slowing the growth of cancer cells, which grow and divide quickly.

The disadvantages are that chemotherapy not only kills fast-growing cancer cells, but also kills or slows the growth of healthy cells that grow and divide quickly. Examples are cells that line your mouth and intestines and those that cause your hair to grow. Damage to healthy cells may cause side effects, such as mouth sores, nausea, and hair loss. The most common side effect is fatigue, a feeling of being exhausted and worn out.

Immunotherapy

Immunotherapy is a type of cancer treatment that helps your immune system fight cancer. It is a biological therapy that uses substances made from living organisms to treat cancer.

The most common side effects are skin reactions at the needle site, such as pain, swelling, rash and itchiness. There can be flu-like symptoms such as fever, weakness, dizziness, nausea, muscle aches, fatigue, headache, shortness of breath and low or high blood pressure. Other side effects might include swelling and weight gain from retaining fluid, heart palpitations, sinus congestion, diarrhoea and risk of infection.

Targeted therapy

Targeted therapy is the foundation of precision medicine. It is a treatment that targets the changes in cancer cells that help them grow, divide and spread. It helps the immune system destroy cancer cells and stop cancer cells growing.

Drawbacks include the fact that cancer cells can become resistant to them, and there are common side effects such as diarrhoea and liver problems.

Other side effects might include problems with blood clotting and wound healing, high blood pressure, fatigue, mouth sores, nail changes, the loss of hair colour and skin problems, including a rash or dry skin. Very rarely, a hole might form through the wall of the oesophagus, stomach, small intestine, large bowel, rectum or gallbladder.

Hormone therapy

Hormone therapy slows or stops the growth of cancers that use hormones to grow. It lessens the chance the cancer will return or stop/slow its growth. It can also ease cancer symptoms.

It can, however, block the body's ability to produce hormones or interfere with the normal hormonal processes. Common side effects for men who receive hormone therapy for prostate cancer include hot flushes, loss of interest in sex, weakened bones, diarrhoea, nausea, enlarged breasts and fatigue. Common side effects for women who receive hormone therapy for breast cancer include hot flushes, vaginal dryness, changes in periods, loss of interest in sex, nausea, fatigue and mood changes.

Stem cell transplant

High doses of chemotherapy or radiation therapy can destroy blood-forming stem cells. Stem cell transplants are procedures that restore these important cells which grow into different types of blood cells. The main types of blood cells are white blood cells which are part of your immune system and help your body fight infection, red blood cells which carry oxygen throughout your body and platelets which help the blood clot.

There are risks to this treatment. The high doses of cancer treatment received before a stem cell transplant can cause problems such as bleeding and an increased risk of infection. If you have an allogeneic transplant, you might develop a serious problem called graft versus host disease (GvHD). This can occur when white blood cells from your donor (the graft) recognize cells in your body (the host) as foreign and attack them. This can damage your skin, liver, intestines and other organs. It can occur weeks after the transplant or much later. GvHD can be treated with steroids or other drugs.[7]

Survival rates

According to Cancer Research UK, there are improvements in some rates of cancer as well as in some survival rates.[8]

Improvement rates

Survival for most cancer types is improving. This progress can generally be attributed to faster diagnosis and advances in treatment. However, there is still scope for improvement and some cancers have shown very little improvement since the early 1970s.

Current versus past survival rates

Prostate cancer has shown the largest improvement in age-standardized ten-year net survival since the early 1970s, from 25 per cent in 1971/1972 to 84 per cent in 2010/2011 (an absolute survival difference of almost 60 percentage points). However, interpretation of survival trends for prostate cancer is made difficult as the types of prostate cancers diagnosed have changed over time due to prostate-specific antigen (PSA) testing. The next largest increases in ten-year survival are for malignant melanoma, non-Hodgkin lymphoma and leukaemia. Bowel cancer and female breast cancer have also shown large improvements in survival over the last 40 years. There has been very little improvement in age-standardized ten-year net survival since the early 1970s for the four lowest surviving cancers in men and women: cancers of the brain, oesophagus, and lung have all shown absolute increases of less than 10 percentage points since 1971/1972, while pancreatic cancer has had no change.

Global deaths from cancer

The most common causes of cancer death worldwide have changed little over the last 40 years. Lung, liver, stomach and bowel cancers have been the four most common causes of cancer death since 1975.

3

Mind and body

The mind–body split

For centuries in the history of medicine it was thought that the mind and body were two separate entities that had little influence on each other. However, in more recent years there has been a shift in recognizing the interconnectedness of the two and how one not only influences and impacts the other but can directly alter its structure and process.

Medical professionals you have seen may not have given this much consideration when you have met with them. If they have, they may have discussed them as though they are two different matters with little or no relationship.

The truth is that the two dimensions are intimately interconnected as we are one entity, mind and body, not two disconnected components. Consequently, it is essential to take care of both your body and your mind simultaneously, and to recognize where they interact.

It is helpful knowing what to expect both physically and psychologically. Guidelines and information are essential for keeping your anxious, fearful self contained. You need to know the physical sensations that might occur, for how long, whom to speak to, when and where. Being aware of how your mood might be affected, your state of mind and your emotional relationships all give you foreknowledge of what might happen.

When there is so much uncertainty and confusion, as well as new symptoms or difficult-to-manage symptoms, there is always the worry that you are being a nuisance asking questions, but whoever is responsible for your care should inform you of what is to be expected and when to call for advice.

Later in the book there are sections on how to take care of your physical body, such as through sleep and exercise, but it is important to take care of your emotional and mental health too by being kind to yourself, using breathing practices on a regular basis, establishing support systems and recognizing the loneliness you may feel. There may be people around you, but illness can evoke powerful feelings of loneliness, either because of poor support systems or as a consequence of facing such a frightening experience that may, for some, nudge you to see your own mortality in a more urgent way.

Take a moment to consider your posture as you sit and read this book, walk around the house or go about your daily routine. When you feel distressed or low you may have a tendency to slump in a chair, to move more slowly, to look down and have a hunched posture. If you are anxious you may sit on the edge of a chair, move quickly and restlessly, fiddle nervously with objects or be unable to sit still for any length of time. Emotional pain can often affect your posture in the same way as physical pain, leading you to adopt defensive or tense positions. On the other hand, when you are confident and calm your shoulders will be back, you will stand up straight and look ahead while walking purposefully, or sit comfortably in a chair in an upright, open and relaxed manner.

Mindfulness Practice: Adjusting Posture

Sit in a chair in a slumped and hunched position for two minutes. Become aware of your breathing and observe any sensations that come to mind. Can you feel any aches and pains? How is it affecting your breathing? What emotions can you identify?

Now sit up straighter with your shoulders back. Your posture should be open and relaxed; try to soften your facial muscles and jaw, and nurture a feeling of confidence and calm. As you continue to focus on your breathing, notice any changes that occur either physically or emotionally. Do you feel more alert, more confident or less anxious? If no changes occur, that is fine too.

Make a mental note of your experience and throughout the day become aware of your posture when you feel anxious or distressed. At these times gently and kindly adjust it if you are hunched, on the edge of your seat or sitting restlessly. Take a moment to think how these small changes may affect your physical and emotional well-being.

Research has shown that not only do your emotions affect your posture but your posture can also affect your emotions.[1] By adjusting your posture you can lift your mood, reduce aches and pains, improve blood flow around the body and increase your energy levels.

The Biopsychosocial Model

The Biopsychosocial Model influences the mind/body perspective. It is the foundation of who you are and why you react and respond to your life experiences, especially in difficult times such as having cancer.

The Biopsychosocial Model[2] is essentially the idea that your biological, psychological and social make-up interact throughout your life. All three elements are important in forming who you are and how you see the world, and each should be considered in relation to the others, thinking about how they interact and influence each other.

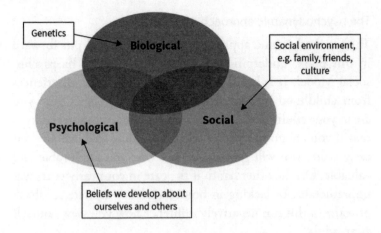

You inherit most of your physical attributes and many of your psychological attributes from your parents through your genes, however it is your experiences which shape your development. Take for example the process of growing a flower in a pot. All of the plant's biological predispositions are contained within the seed that you plant, but its growth and characteristics will also be affected by how often you water it, the quality of the soil, how much sunlight it receives and other factors. In a similar way, humans inherit traits from their parents but their environments and experiences, particularly during early development, lay the foundations for their psychological and emotional make-up which will influence their decisions and choices throughout their lives.

All three elements – biological, psychological and social – contribute to who you are today and have influenced your perception of the world and your choices, whether consciously or unconsciously.

The psychodynamic approach

The psychodynamic approach, within the model put forward in this book, underpins the 'psycho' part of the Biopsychosocial Model. It is based on the theory that your experiences from childhood into adulthood considerably affect who you are in your adult years and how you act. The common theory is that if you are given regular, reliable and engaged care in your early years, you will grow to believe that you are lovable and valuable. On the other hand, if the care in your early years was unpredictable or lacking in boundaries, appropriate feedback or warmth this can negatively influence how you view yourself as an adult.[3]

Biological, psychological, social and early-life experiences are intricately linked and who you are today is a result of every experience you have had up to this point – the wonderful, the boring and the horrible. You have learned to survive and have many internal resources that work to your benefit. However, through life you may also have developed ways of protecting yourself, for example, not asking for help so you won't be disappointed if it isn't there, or thinking you will be a nuisance if you tell others you are in pain. These protective shields usually develop early in life, particularly through your experiences with your caregivers. They can sometimes get in the way of managing difficult life situations, such as cancer, and affect your relationships or quality of life. Becoming more aware of, and alert to, these factors can help you gain perspective on how you relate to yourself and others. It can help you to gain a clearer picture of what fits where, make sense of it and place it within a context.[4]

Below is a short task. It can help you to think about how the different parts of the Biopsychosocial Model and your own personal dynamics interact and impact on your current situation and life in general. Draw a table like Table 1 below and use it to identify the different aspects of each area that are pertinent to you.

Table 1

Biological	Psychological	Social	Early experiences

Now use the information you put into Table 1 and link it to the sections outlined in Table 2 below.

Table 2

How they affect me?	How they affect my relationships with professionals?	How they affect my social and family relationships?	How they impact on my illness and its management?

4

Mindfulness, meditation and cancer

A mindful approach

Mindfulness is not relaxation, trying to empty your mind of your anxieties or a therapy that will cure your cancer. Rather, it is a way of developing your internal resources, resilience and balance, which can help you to deal with life's challenges and your response to them. It can help you to hold onto the good that is still around you and to develop a way of managing your distress so that you feel more in control of it and of the events in your life.

It's about paying attention to what is happening within you and around you, in this moment, without criticism or judgement, and to be with your thoughts, feelings and responses without the need to reject or change them.

Key points about mindfulness

- It is an approach to life which involves both practices and developing a way of being – a mindset.
- It can be developed and used by anyone, when appropriate.
- It is about encouraging your ability to be open to this moment of time for whatever it brings.
- It is not about achieving relaxation or an altered state of mind.
- It is a resource you can draw on in difficult times and a way to fully enjoy the good times.

History of mindfulness

Mindfulness and meditation have become secularized from their original roots in Buddhism and other contemplative philosophies.[1] Meditations focusing on breathing and being present in the moment are an important part of Buddhist practices, and their effectiveness and usefulness have filtered through to the Western world over the centuries. In 1979, Jon Kabat-Zinn and his colleagues at the University of Massachusetts developed a programme that integrated these mindfulness practices into a structured format to provide interventions for people suffering from physical and emotional distress in a hospital setting. This programme became known as Mindfulness-Based Stress Reduction (MBSR), and is now an internationally recognized programme used worldwide for a variety of physical and emotional conditions.

Mindfulness Practice: Breathe and Observe

- Breathe into your distress.
- Breathe into the centre of the distress.
- Breathe and release.
- Breathe and observe what is happening.
- Notice the tension in your body where the distress sits.
- Notice the tension in your body around the distress and beyond it.
- Simply observe it.
- Breathe and observe.
- How far does it extend?
- Where is the pain, physical or emotional?
- Breathe and observe what is happening.
- Breathe – observe – breathe – release – breathe.

Mindfulness is not about avoiding what you are experiencing; it's about taming your emotions and your thoughts. Just because you think something doesn't mean it's true. You were feeling lucky last Saturday – did you have that winning lottery ticket?

Research on how mindfulness can help with cancer

There has been a plethora of research over the past few years into mindfulness and its benefits for cancer symptoms. Below are a few research outcomes that you may find of interest, although this is only the tip of the iceberg.

Stress reduction

- In a review of nine research articles and five conference abstracts, mostly conducted with breast and prostate cancer patients, improved psychological function was consistently found through practising a mindfulness intervention in a clinic-based group.[2]
- 27 women diagnosed with breast cancer showed significant decreases in stress and state anxiety levels. Also results showed significant and beneficial changes for mental adjustment to cancer and health locus of control (HLOC) scores following completion of the MBSR intervention.[3]

Psychosocial adjustment

- MBSR may improve cancer patients' psychosocial adjustment to their disease.[4]

Enhanced coping

- It appears that learning how to be mindful is beneficial for women after their treatment for breast cancer. In women who had received breast cancer treatment, adherence to an MBSR programme resulted in 91 per cent of participants experiencing significant improvements in coping with the illness, and significant reductions in stress, depression and medical symptoms.[5]

Sexual functioning

- 13 research papers and four conference abstracts published since 2007 reported five different types of mindfulness intervention. The studies reported significant improvements in sexual difficulties and physiological arousal across all interventions.[6]

Quality of life

- Mindfulness meditation was found to improve quality of life for cancer outpatients and these improvements were maintained three months later.[7]
- Individuals with head and neck cancer showed an association between higher post-intervention mindfulness and higher total, social and emotional quality of life after completing an MBSR programme when undergoing curative treatment.[8]

Pain

- Mindfulness-Based Cognitive Therapy (MBCT) showed a significant and durable beneficial effect on pain intensity in women treated for primary breast cancer.[9]
- Pain self-efficacy and expressive suppression improved significantly for women with breast cancer after three weeks of a mindfulness intervention.[10]

Mood disturbance

- Breast cancer survivors had significantly lower levels of depression, anxiety and fear of cancer recurrence after completing an MBSR course when compared with patients in usual care.[11]

- An MBSR programme for cancer outpatients was effective in decreasing mood disturbance and stress symptoms for up to six months in both male and female patients with a variety of cancer diagnoses, stages of illness and educational background.[12]
- Participating in a weekly 90-minute meditation group for seven weeks with home practice in between sessions effectively lowered mood disturbance and stress symptoms in cancer outpatients.[13]

Energy

- A group of breast cancer survivors had higher energy levels after completing MBSR compared with those following usual care.[14]
- An MBSR programme for breast cancer survivors improved fatigue, drowsiness, emotional well-being, quality of life, stress, anxiety and depression after six weeks. The effects did not improve further after 12 weeks, however they were sustained.[15]

Sleep quality

- Three randomized controlled clinical trials and seven uncontrolled clinical trials were conducted. Studies reported positive results such as improved sleep quality, mood and stress reduction.[16]

Immune system

- Women with breast cancer receiving MBSR (eight weekly group sessions) saw significant benefits in immune function, as well as significant improvements in depression, symptom burden, distress and mental health.[17, 18]

How can mindfulness help?

There are some key points to note about mindfulness and mindfulness meditations or practices. A central aspect of mindfulness is that everything in life is transient; it is impermanent. By developing and enhancing your focus, you become aware of how there are fluctuations in each moment of your existence. Your feelings and thoughts shift, your physical discomfort shifts, your situation shifts and with each moment of life comes an altered perception. You notice the subtle nuances of change by observing and focusing.

Mindfulness enhances your focus, concentration and awareness and by so doing it develops your ability to gather your energies to attend to a specific experience. This awareness and focused energy helps you to move towards your distress so that you can examine its location, intensity and variations, your response to it and how others respond to it. It opens up the possibility for you to respond to your situation not with fear and rejection but with a kindness and sense of control.

Mindfulness develops your ability and capacity to both experience what is happening to you, including the good things and not only your illness, as well as view it from above or from a step removed. It gives you a meta view and perspective. Meta means beyond, so this process involves thinking beyond your thoughts, feeling beyond your feelings and so forth. It is you having the experience and an awareness of the process of how you think, feel and respond to that experience. This is not disassociating or cutting off from an experience.

Metacognition

The ability to think about your thinking is what neuroscientists call metacognition. It refers to the process of stepping back to see what you are doing, being an observer, watching and noticing your responses. Metacognition involves two distinct but interrelated areas – metacognitive knowledge and metacognitive regulation or control. Metacognitive knowledge involves awareness of your thinking, knowledge of yourself as a learner, knowledge of the aspects of the task and strategies needed to carry it out. Metacognitive regulation involves your ability to manage your thinking processes, which strategies you actually use in order to make cognitive progress such as planning your approach to a task, evaluating its progress and, importantly, being able to change tactics or direction if there are difficulties.[19]

It is about developing awareness of what you think, do, feel and believe when you go through an experience. It's like seeing a daffodil as a whole flower but also being able to recognize that there are different parts of it (the petals, their colour variations, the stem, the stamen, the stalk and leaves) that can be separate but that come together to form the flower. This awareness of the process of how these parts work both separately and together don't make the daffodil any less of a flower or alter it in any way; it simply gives you a greater knowledge and perspective of it.

Mindfulness develops your capacity for, and draws on, metacognitive knowledge and metacognitive regulation. As interest in mindfulness has grown significantly in recent years, there has been an increasing number of research studies investigating the potential benefits of mindfulness on the symptoms of cancer, with only a few mentioned in this chapter.

Focused attention

Meditation, within the context of mindfulness, refers to paying attention to the present moment, without judgement, for whatever it is. By focusing on your breathing, the most automatic of functions, in this moment without evaluating or judging it, you are able to appreciate and absorb the moment for what it is; the sensations in your body, the sights, sounds and smells around you, the emotions you are experiencing, in a stable, balanced and focused way. You notice and observe rather than comment on or judge it.

Thoughts

We take our thoughts for granted and believe each one that comes to us. However, we need to turn the idea of thoughts on its head as thoughts are not concrete, proven facts. They are transient things that we hold onto and to which we give enormous power. We don't have to. They can shift, move, change, dissipate and even disappear. Alternatively, if we insist on focusing so much energy on them, they can grow and breed into dense, strangling jungles.

Through mindfulness, you will get to experience how you can step aside from the jungle and into a different mindset where a more gentle and caring space nurtures you in your own mind. Meditation provides stillness or at least quiet, even if only for a moment in time. One moment, and perhaps another, and another.

Mindfulness may assist on occasions, but the real value will be felt if you immerse yourself in the practices, doing them on a regular, daily basis if possible. However, it's not only about the practices but the philosophy and mindset of it. Perhaps one of the most helpful aspects of a mindful mindset is recognizing that life is, by its very nature, transient and impermanent: it shifts, changes, adapts and moves on, just like your thoughts. Clinging on to situations or experiences (which is a natural thing to do especially if they are good, loving and keep you alive) and imagining that you can keep them static and the same forever only leads to suffering. More on this later.

Mindfulness takes on a particular value when you let it become your companion. Sometimes it will be annoying, but it will always be there to support you and to hold your hand when you feel fearful, alone or want to laugh at the ironies of life. When you feel a deep sense of something, such as pain, fear or sadness, let it be there, stay with it, breathe and breathe into it, and it will soften. Not disappear or be removed but soften.

Mindfulness Practice: A Moment of Stillness

This exercise is a simple but effective way to begin to understand what mindfulness is about. It can be used as a starting point or as a marker of your progress as you become more involved in the process of mindfulness.

- Sit in stillness for two minutes.

- Pay attention to what thoughts and sensations are going through your mind and body. Is there an itch in your leg? Have you just remembered that you need to pay the phone bill? Do your shoulders feel tense? Is your heart pounding? Are you thinking about all the things on your 'to do' list?

What was it like sitting in stillness? Did you feel comfortable or were you in any physical or emotional discomfort? Did you start to feel calmer or did your anxiety start to increase? Did the time go quickly or slowly? Why do you think that was?

In times of crisis, it is hard to believe that anything other than practical interventions can have much value. The tests and treatments, the appointments and decisions take precedence over emotional needs. During this time, and at the same time as all the practical matters need to be addressed, let the universe hold you, let your breath be your anchor, your compass and your most valued and precious force. Let it nourish you and it will give you a sense of control and power to tether yourself in the moments of quiet and when storms hit. It will heal and comfort, not the cancer, but what comes with it physically and emotionally.

Important note: By starting to engage more with your thoughts and by understanding the events that have brought you to where you are now, feelings and memories may be brought to the fore which could be painful or upsetting. Should this happen, be aware of the sensation but manage it in a positive way, by listening to music or talking to a friend, for example. If the feelings are very distressing, you should seek the input of a qualified professional. Therapy should not be regarded as embarrassing or intimidating; it is simply two people coming together to explore your life and develop your understanding of these feelings to better deal with them.

Scepticism is fine

Being sceptical about this approach is fine and to be expected. If you are unfamiliar with the ideas and concepts put forward in this book, read on with an open mind and see what happens. If you find it's too much or not currently of interest to you, skim through or put it to one side for another time. There really is no expectation that you will take to this approach or find it of interest. If you don't like it, dump it. You have enough to contend with.

With mindfulness the benefits come from both your approach and continuing to do the practices – without them it's like taking half your dose of medication and then wondering why it's not helping or stopping it because you think it's ineffective. Mindfulness isn't just for today or this week; it's a resource that you develop within yourself with each observation, with each practice, with each experience. It becomes your anchor that you can drop when the seas get rough or you simply want to remain calm and steady in shifting times.

It's an ongoing process that happens gradually. It takes time, effort, trial and error, and ongoing engagement. It takes a willingness to be open to a different experience, to a way of observing your illness, the emotions around it and other aspects of your life without any specific purpose other than to observe and be open to them, with kindness. Through this, your relationship to your illness and its effects, and to yourself, will begin to shift.

5

I might have cancer, I do have cancer

Being diagnosed with cancer is a real shock and it is often that sense of shock, that experience when being told, that stays with you.

There are so many feelings associated with a diagnosis, its treatment and outcome.

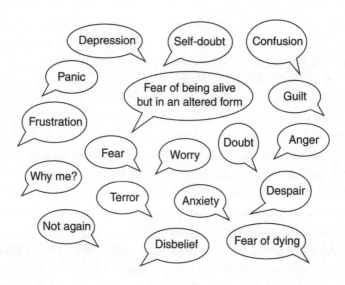

Added to this are the feelings that come from treatment and needing help from others, such as fatigue, feeling vulnerable, being dependent, sadness, grief, loss, longing, stress and exhaustion.

Having cancer can be overwhelming, all-consuming, daunting and terrifying.

A change in dynamics

Having cancer is like being caught up in a tsunami. A diagnosis evokes complex, complicated, confusing and contradictory dynamics and emotions. This includes a dynamic between you and medical professionals. You need to work out what to trust and who to trust. There is also the dynamic that develops between you and those around you – your family, friends, support workers and so on. Are they rescuers, intruders, helpers?

Sometimes you need to shut down in order to manage the flood of emotions, decisions, procedures and interventions. Everyone will approach this in their own way but often in line with your own perspective, attitude and mindset. If you have always been a structured, controlled, organized and informed person then you will probably be the same through your illness. Others may rely on professionals and look to them to make decisions if that is the way they have been throughout most of their lives up until now.

Trust and making decisions

When you are faced with such a crisis and you don't know which route to take or what the outcome will be, who to trust becomes a big issue. Trust as it covers a wide range of people and issues such professionals, procedures and interventions, advice, treatments and the support of others. The most important factor is that you need to know, and believe in, what is true for you regarding your needs, your wishes and your treatment. You might need to negotiate with others, make difficult decisions, decide to make changes or reorganize your work, home, lifestyle or some other factor.

Remember, it's your body, your life, your choice.

If you feel you are making a decision or choice that doesn't fit in with what others believe or want, you might feel guilty. Others may even threaten to reject you or distance themselves from you for this but that is their choice. You have a right to do what you want with your body and your life. You have a choice about the decisions you make. You can consider others and review the options, but you must be honest with yourself and true to yourself so that you have a real idea of what it is you want for your life, your illness, your body and your future.

It can be easier said than done, but know that whatever you decide is the result of you being true to yourself. It's hard to avoid asking 'what if', but once you have made a decision don't second guess the outcome, look back or play out every possible scenario. If you keep changing your mind or over-think the decision you have made, you will be riddled with self-doubt, confusion and anxiety.

Mindfulness can help you with your need for an answer. As you allow the internal noise in your head to be present but not intrusive, you can permit a quiet within and it is in those quiet moments or seconds that the seed of your decision will begin to grow and present itself.

In terms of trust, you may feel too scared to surrender to anything, but it is important to allow yourself to take what is being offered and let it in even if you are unsure, sceptical, cynical or scared. When you commit all of yourself to something it becomes easier and more satisfying because doubt and criticism sap your will and energy. Open your heart to what is happening even though your impulse is to shut yourself off, to withdraw, hide and swaddle yourself in layers of protection.

Mindfulness Practice: A Moment of Calm in Two Minutes

This two-minute breathing practice is an excellent introduction to how focusing on your breathing can help to settle and ground you. It is particularly useful when your chest or stomach feels tight, your heart is pounding or you are feeling bombarded by distressing thoughts. It can be done at any time and in any place when you feel off balance or anxious: before, during or after treatment; while waiting for an appointment; during the day or night when fear or sadness strike or after a difficult conversation. It can also be used if you have returned to work, maybe while you are in the staff room (or even the toilet if necessary) or in those moments when you are feeling overwhelmed.

- Sit in a chair with your eyes open or closed and place one hand on your stomach, feeling it rise and fall. Without forcing your breath in any way, silently count 'in, 2, 3, 4' on the inbreath and 'out, 2, 3, 4' on the outbreath. Repeat this three times.

- Breathe in for the same amount of time as above, but count only 'in, 2, 3' on the inbreath and 'out, 2, 3' on the outbreath. Repeat three times, then reduce it to 'in, 2, out, 2' and repeat three times. Now take one breath in and one breath out, without counting. If this feels difficult, think 'in' and 'out' to the rhythm of your breathing. Repeat three times.

- Take a moment to think about how you feel. Do you feel calmer? Is your breathing more regular? Do you feel less tense and have your physical symptoms of anxiety subsided a little?

- Take this moment of calm with you, knowing that returning to a calmer and more balanced state of mind can be as simple as breathing.

When you take the time to sit in stillness, often your mind starts to fill with thoughts, ruminations, anxieties and fears around your illness. In the following sections the mindfulness practices will help to develop your focus, allowing you to take a step back from these worries. This process involves thinking beyond your thoughts, feeling beyond your feelings – a meta view, as previously mentioned.

Life is like a road trip. It covers many miles over a vast distance and there are multiple phases to it. Your cancer is part of that road trip and one of its phases, and there is no limit to the number of places you will pass by or stop at as your life progresses. There will be sunshine, storms, dust, heat, traffic, open spaces, detours, diversions, magnificent views, frightening or exhausting journeys, and they are all part of your road trip. The aim is to navigate those experiences because if you manage them in some way that is helpful, or at least not destructive, you can cope with those parts that aren't the way you would have liked them to be.

It would be wonderful to say that mindfulness and meditation are the answer to all your problems, that they will ease the emotional and physical distress that comes with cancer, that they will allow you to face the pain and heart ache, the fear and the unknown with ease and without disruption. They won't, but what they can do is help you to develop an approach and a practice that can help nurture you with compassion and kindness while you deal with whatever is happening.

Support

No-one wants the experience of having cancer but by shutting yourself down and barricading your heart from the flood of emotions you are also cutting yourself off from the fact (and joy) that you are alive right now, that people around you care about you, love you and want to be connected to you.

It's unrealistic to think that everyone has a strong and powerful support system around them or that each person has a group of family and friends who will be available. The truth is that some people may only have one or two people in their network, or no-one close enough to rely on or be there for assistance. For those who have fewer sources to draw on, it is about accepting support from organizations or groups, whatever form that may take.

The fantasy is that when we are ill or distressed people will automatically know we are and will naturally be available to help us. This isn't always the case so permit yourself to ask for help, make suggestions about what will help and when, and let people do what they are offering to do. Often it is our pride that gets in the way or our self-esteem – we think we ought to be able to go it alone. Alternatively, we believe that we aren't worthy of help from others (I'll be a nuisance; it's an imposition; they don't know me; it's care from a stranger etc.) and so we reject it even if we want it. Let others be there with you and for you. Often, it's not that they aren't there but that we are reluctant to let them hold our hand in whatever form it is offered.

The other side of this is that others may shut their hearts and minds to what is happening as it can be so fearful and overwhelming for them. They may step back from you, shut down their emotions or distance themselves emotionally or literally.

Ask yourself the following questions:

- Who do you feel safe with?
- What comforts you?
- What supports you?
- Who supports you?

- How do they do it?
- Why do you let them?
- When don't you let them?
- When do you let them?
- Are there others you can't or won't let support or comfort you?
- Why?
- What gets in the way of you asking for help or support?

Tell people what you need – they can't read your mind and what you wanted in the past may not be the same as what you want or need now. Be mindful of others and check what will work for them too. However, you may need to put boundaries around their overprotective approach or attitude. They may have intrusive questions, be constantly worrying and ruminating, or have distressing fears. Telling you this can increase your anxiety or hinder your being able to tell them of your feelings. They may have an overcontrolling or distant manner, or perhaps are unable to speak of their emotions, none of which are helpful to you. Setting boundaries is difficult but during your time of distress it is important that you place a fence around others' expressions or behaviours in order to protect yourself.

We all deal with things in our own way and it may be hard to tell those who love and care for you that they need to contain their emotions or be more engaged with yours. However, it is vital that you use your energy to protect and take care of yourself where you can. The following is a practice to help you focus on your senses while doing a simple daily task.

Mindfulness Practice: The Shower

- While you are in the shower feel the sensation of the drops of water hitting your skin, the warmth of the water relaxing your muscles and invigorating you.

- Open your mouth, let the drops hit your tongue and feel the water running over your lips and chin.

- Relax into this and become aware of the water against the rest of your body and the sensations that come with that.

Only you can walk down this road, alone in its enormity but not necessarily alone in isolation.

6

Fear, worry and anxiety

Fear is a remarkably powerful emotion. It can take over your thinking as well as generate high levels of stress within your mind and body. Much of it comes down to the difference between what you want, crave or desire versus what you have right now. You want health but you have illness; you want stability and certainty but all you have is anxiety and uncertainty; you want to be well but all you have is pain and fear.

Fear can cover many areas and go deep into your psyche. There are some fears that have little to do with your cancer and others that have only emerged since your diagnosis. Some may have been there but were unrecognized or held at bay and now show themselves with force. You could have a fear of:

- who you are
- what you want
- how you feel
- what others think of you – your mind, body and actions
- the unknown
- your illness
- rejection
- intimacy
- vulnerability
- physical contact
- being exposed
- being seen as a fraud
- criticism
- being unwanted

- pain
- risk
- change
- life
- death

Recognizing your fears and being with them can help you to work with them rather than push them out. When you are ill and perhaps facing your mortality for the first time, life takes on a sense of urgency. What was put aside, avoided or repressed may now come to the surface, either with enormous force or in small bits.

Give yourself a time slot to worry. Tell yourself you are not going to worry now but you will do it later.

Worry and fear can become like an addiction (I must have it, do it, I can't live without it, something will happen if I don't worry). Worry, fear, anxiety, depression – they are powerful and can be overwhelming and dominate your existence, and you need to stand up to them. These feelings come from within you, so you can learn to manage the extent of impact they are to have on your daily life.

Am I allowed to feel stillness, quiet, peace or acceptance if I'm ill? Of course, you are going to feel scared, terrified, angry, worried and many other difficult emotions. The issue is what are you going to do with those feelings and how are you going to manage them?

The trick is in the word 'manage' – not avoid, not deny, not dive into, not wallow, not reject, but allow and manage. You can't manage your feelings if you won't allow them. Much of this is made more difficult by us feeling ashamed at what we feel and our less than stoic response, even if that response is only known to ourselves.

An anxious mind

Research in neuroscience, the scientific study of the brain and nervous system, has shown that following a traumatic or frightening event, there are physical changes in the brain caused by the release of neurotransmitters (brain chemicals) that mirror psychological reactions.[1] Neuronal (brain) pathways are created which become stronger each time they are activated. This means that when a strategy is activated, for example, fear and nausea when you walk into a hospital, it strengthens the link between the distressing emotion, the psychological reaction and the pathway set up in your brain. This then increases the likelihood that the next time the emotion is experienced the same reaction will be triggered[2] and the same neuronal pathway activated. Every time you experience that situation or a similar one, your brain immediately puts you onto that pathway without you even having to think about it. The pathways are like railway tracks so if your association puts you on to the track going to London, that's the route you'll take even if you want to go to Wales. The more the pathway is activated the stronger it becomes.

This research shows that not only can we become psychologically conditioned to follow a certain behaviour or defence mechanism to deal with a distressing emotion, but our brains can also physically change as a result, reinforcing the connection between the emotion and the behaviour. An anxious or fearful mind may be predisposed to creating these neuronal pathways more quickly or more deeply, which may account for why anxiety and fear persist long after the event or emotion that triggered it.[3]

The negative bias

Psychologists have established that humans have evolved to have a 'negative bias' in their attention.[4] This means that you attend more to negative events or emotions than those that are neutral or positive because they signify potential threats to you. At an evolutionary level, you are wired to quickly notice and identify anything that may harm you, allowing you to respond as rapidly as possible.[5] However, this negative bias is also one of the reasons that you sometimes form stronger memories of upsetting experiences than pleasant ones or tend to focus on the negative aspects of situations. A strong negative bias is one of the underlying reasons behind anxious and fearful thoughts which give rise to feelings of nervousness, apprehension or despair.[6] This may contribute to your distress as it can be difficult to concentrate on the easier or happier moments so life looks bleak.

Needless to say, when faced with an illness or negative experience such as having cancer, there is a realistic swing towards the negative as you don't know the outcome and the treatment interventions can be harsh and frightening, sometimes having long-lasting side effects or consequences.

What becomes important in this situation is that the swing towards the negative doesn't dominate to the extent that all or any positive is blackened over or stifled. This is where mindfulness can come into play. By doing the practices on a regular basis, it can help balance the impact of an ongoing negative bias and prevent or soften the extent of development of the brain pathways that can take you into very dark places in your head. A practice as simple as the one below (body focus) can bring about a powerful shift in your focus and your increased stress level evoked by your emotions or thoughts.

Mindfulness can help to give you a new way of managing your life despite feeling such distress.

Body focus

When someone is physically ill, their body becomes the focus of many emotions. With something like cancer, you want to get rid of it, and you may feel alienated from your body as you start to view it differently when it is the source of distress and fear, and full of unpleasant or strange sensations. At times, you may want to reject your body because of all that is happening physically and emotionally. You will be poked and prodded a lot and this increases as treatment progresses. The physical reactions to treatment such as chemotherapy can leave you feeling disgusted or fearful of any bodily sensation or response. A paradox is set up as you hate the body that is ill but cling to every breath that it allows, and you desperately want it to heal.

In a positive way, this body focus practice helps you to reconnect to the body that you have lost faith in. It reminds you that there are various parts that make up your physical existence in the world and that they all require attention and care. It is important because illness, pain and discomfort can distort your beliefs about yourself as well as your body. This practice encourages you to recognize where the primary discomfort or sensation is occurring, its location, quality and intensity, and where other parts of your body may be affected as an extension of the primary source of illness. In addition to this, you start to realize that there are parts of your body, no matter if it is only a hand or finger, that are working well. By paying attention to your body in the specific manner of this practice, it will help to remind you that your body is one whole made up of many parts and that they are vitally interconnected.

Mindfulness Practice: Body Focus

🔊 Find a quiet place to carry out this practice. Switch your phone to silent or leave it in another room. Ask others around you not to disturb you unless it is an emergency. Wear comfortable clothing and make sure that you will be warm enough – perhaps have a blanket nearby as your body temperature will drop. This is also an excellent practice for physical pain.

- Choose a position which is comfortable and works well for you (see the diagrams below). The ideal position is lying flat on your back on the floor, on a rug or blanket if there is no carpet, with a cushion for your head if this increases your comfort.

- Use any cushions, blankets or other supports that help you to be comfortable.

- Place your legs on a chair, straight or bent, if that is easier on your back. An alternative is lying on a bed, especially if you have difficulty getting to the floor. If lying down is uncomfortable or difficult for you, you can sit in a chair which provides sufficient support, using footstools or cushions to ensure your comfort. If sitting is not ideal, you can stand or lean against a wall, ensuring you have a steady object to lean upon (see diagrams below).

- A note about breathing: When the track says 'breathe into your toes' or any other part of your body, it is meant metaphorically. Physiologically we are unable to breathe into any part of our body other than our lungs, so it is about imagining the breath moving through your body. By placing your breath into an area of your body in your imagination, you are bringing attention and focus to it and relaxing the area.

- Before starting the practice, take a moment to think about how you are feeling. Take note of any physical sensations of stress or anxiety, as well as any thoughts or emotions that are at the forefront of your mind. Tell yourself that this is very important for your psychological and physical well-being.

Listen to the body focus practice which you will find in the audio file accompanying this book.

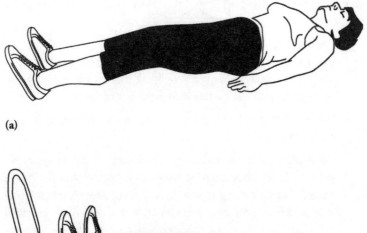

(a)

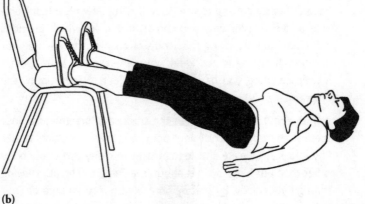

(b)

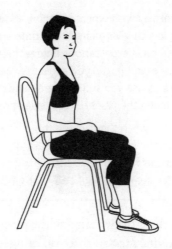

(c)

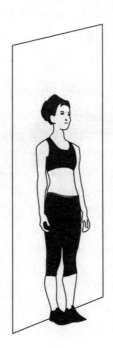

(d)

After the practice, take a few moments to think about your response to it before moving. Did you give yourself the time and space to do the practice? What were your expectations before the practice, and were they reasonable? For example, did you expect to feel much calmer but now feel frustrated because you still feel tense and stressed? Were you cynical at first, but found the practice enjoyable and relaxing?

Most people fall asleep when they first do this practice. However, if you find that you continually fall asleep when doing it, it is helpful to do it sitting up until you can remain alert throughout. The purpose of the practice is to bring awareness to your body not send you off to sleep.

A written sample of the wording of the practice can be found below. It has been included so that you can get an idea of what it is about and be reassured that there is nothing in any of the practices that aims to put you into a trance-like or altered state of mind. All you are doing is breathing.

Sample transcript from the body focus practice

The intention is to bring awareness to the different parts of the body without moving or stretching them in any way. It is about experiencing the sensations within your body, making no demands on it.

As you breathe in and out, become aware that this is your body, all of it, for whatever it is: the parts that work well and keep you alive, and the part that are damaged and in pain.

Now focus on the big toe of your left foot. Become aware of the existence of this part of your body and the sensations that might be there. Let your attention go deep into the toe, not moving it, just observing it and feeling whatever is or isn't happening in it at this moment. If you feel no sensations that too is fine. Simply acknowledge whatever is there.

Now move your focus to the little toe on the left foot – and to all the toes. Become aware of the feelings within the toes, acknowledge them, and breathe deep into the toes on an inbreath. And on an out-breath let go of your awareness of the toes, letting their existence drift and dissolve from your mind.

Now bring your attention to the sole of your left foot, focusing on any sensations deep within the foot, aware of the air against it, your instep, the heel against the floor. Breathing in and out of it and on the outbreath let go of your awareness of it and bring it to the top of the left foot, becoming familiar with the sensations in this part of your body, of all the small bones that make up the foot. Breathing all the way into it, and then on an outbreath letting it dissolve from awareness.

Moving your focus to the left ankle, feeling and acknowledging what-ever it is that is there, aware of the bones that come together to form a joint. Breathing into it and out of it, letting it go. Now focus on the foot and ankle as a whole, breathing deep into it. Let your breath travel, in your mind's eye, all the way down from the nostrils, through the chest and abdomen, down the left leg and into the foot and an-kle, aware of the oxygen coming to it and when it gets there, release and let the breath travel all the way back out through the nostrils and on an outbreath let the foot and ankle dissolve from your awareness.

Remember, the practices are there to help you to switch on, not to switch off.

7

Stress

All the steps involved in getting a diagnosis and having treatment can create an enormous amount of stress and stressful situations that may continue for many years. Understanding how your mind and body react to stress and the implications of it are important as it can become detrimental to your well-being. Consequently, it is important to find ways of managing and containing your stress levels. The research on mindfulness has shown its well-proven benefits in this area and for other factors, such as quality of life and fatigue for those with cancer, as previously noted.

More evidence

New brain imaging technologies have enabled psychologists and neuroscientists to study the effects of mindfulness in new and advanced ways. Functional magnetic resonance imaging (fMRI) scans can give precise visual indications of changes in brain structure before and after adopting mindfulness practices, as well as comparing the brains of people who practise mindfulness and those who don't.

The research shows that mindfulness meditation can:

- increase the brain's grey matter in areas responsible for regulating emotions, sensations and thoughts[1]
- increase impulse control[2] and improve reasoning and decision-making skills[3]

- improve executive functions such as memory and attention[4]
- decrease stress and levels of stress hormones, improve quality of life, improve mood, decrease levels of depression and reduce the effects of trauma[5]
- improve quality of sleep, promote a sense of happiness and improve relationship satisfaction.[6]

It is effective not only for dealing with stress but for dealing with many of the issues facing people who have a physical illness, as well as the emotional concerns that may arise from the illness. A fundamental element of mindfulness practice is that it reduces the stress response, and considering the anxieties and fears associated with having cancer, it is useful to become familiar with how the stress response works in order to work with it in your daily life.

Stress is a biological and psychological response experienced on encountering a threat, whether that threat be real or perceived to be real. Your body's response to stress is a primitive, automatic mechanism to ensure your survival. It is activated at the smallest hint of danger and is always on alert for any threatening situation.

Your brain cannot distinguish between the different types of stressful or distressing situations that occur in life. It doesn't know that the tension you feel when you are distressed or in pain is different from you being in a potentially life-threatening situation. It interprets both as one and the same thing – it thinks you are in danger even if you are not. You being distressed and reacting to it is perceived as a potential threat to your survival, and this is what is referred to as a perceived threat because you aren't actually in immediate danger in the way you would be if a lion jumped out at you.

Your brain kicks into gear at any actual or perceived signal of danger. A threat sets off a physiological reaction via the sympathetic nervous system which switches you to 'go' mode. Once the threat has passed, your body should return to its normal state. The method of the body returning to its normal state is via the parasympathetic system which puts you back to 'rest' mode.

Table 3

Sympathetic system – go mode	Parasympathetic system – rest mode
Adrenalin and cortisol are released into blood	Noradrenalin is released into blood
Breathing rate increases	Breathing rate decreases
Heart rate levels rise	Heart rate levels lower
Energy is directed to heart, muscles and lungs Digestive process shuts down	Energy is redirected to other organs in the body that help with digestion, absorption, excretion and other essential functions

When stress is continually experienced, your sympathetic nervous system remains in a more active state than it needs to be. This phenomenon is extremely important because over time this can bring about both physical and psychological problems as your mind and body become exhausted.

Consequences of non-stop stress

There is known to be a link (an association but not necessarily a cause-and-effect response) between stress and multiple conditions such as the following.

- Damage to organs and memory cells
- Distorted thinking
- Fatty deposits around waist
- Irritable bowel syndrome (IBS)
- Aging
- Depression
- Hypertension
- Anxiety/panic attacks
- Heart disease
- Rheumatoid arthritis
- Diabetes
- Cancer
- Pain conditions
- Sleep
- Infertility
- Impotence
- Loss of libido
- Relationship difficulties
- Work performance
- Decrease in quality of life

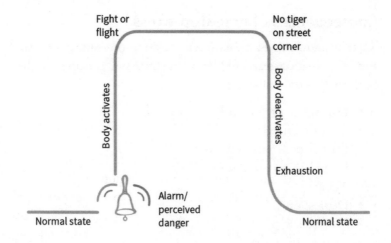

(a)

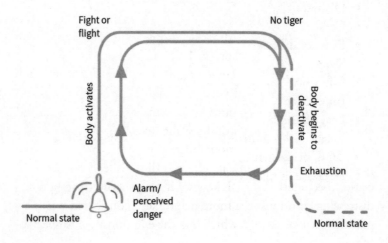

(b)

Intercepting the stress response

Mindfulness has been shown to have a positive effect on the brain because the practices and approach can intercept the stress response before it has damaging effects from unnecessary activation.[7] That is not to say that by practising mindfulness you will never be stressed or have feelings of fear, anxiety or helplessness, especially considering that you have cancer. Rather, by developing a mindful approach to life, you will be able to deal with distressing or fearful situations as they arise, preventing the chronic exposure to stress hormones that can cause the physical problems and mental exhaustion previously discussed. In addition, mindfulness may help to regulate release of neurotransmitters and increase the number of connections between different areas of the brain.[7] These physical changes in the brain then give rise to improved function which can influence your emotional state.

The brain is an extraordinarily complex and fascinating organ as it has the ability to adapt, grow and change according to your experiences. Although neural pathways may be made between distressing emotions and your psychological processes, you can choose to shift your reactions by learning to respond in a different way. Through the mindfulness meditations, you can alter the way you process information and respond to it. When a neural pathway is activated less, its effect is diminished and the association becomes weaker. Likewise, if you choose to respond to distressing emotions in a more helpful and considered way, new pathways will be created which link the emotions to positive coping mechanisms.[8]

Remember, what fires together wires together so the more you criticize yourself or focus on fear or the unknown future, the stronger that pathway becomes. Soften your approach to yourself and your situation and you will not only lessen the strength of those pathways but begin to develop new, more positive ones when you recognize and reinforce a more balanced view of yourself and the life that you have right now. Below is a mindfulness practice that encourages you to engage with your sense of taste.

Mindfulness Practice: Mindful Eating

- Take a piece of fruit, chocolate or any other food which is not too difficult to chew.

- Eat one piece as normal.

- Now take another piece of food, place it on your tongue and let it sit there for a few moments.

- Bring all of your attention to the sensation in your mouth as you let the food remain in your mouth without chewing or swallowing it. What does it feel like in your mouth? Rough or smooth? What does it taste like and can you identify any elements to the taste that you had not noticed on the previous piece?

- Chew the food slowly. What other sensations do you feel? Is it difficult to resist the urge to swallow? Now swallow and notice the movements that come with this action.

8

Mindful awareness

The importance of breathing

Much of the effectiveness of mindfulness can be traced back to its emphasis on the most basic of functions – breathing. Breathing is essential for survival, but it also plays a key role in the management of stress. Most people have heard the idea of taking deep breaths in order to calm down. Although everyone instinctively knows how to breathe, we do not necessarily know how to breathe well. We tend to breathe into the shallowest part of our lungs which have the least flexibility and space. The effect of this is that the amount of air entering our lungs is reduced, and the pattern of our breathing is shallow and irregular.

If you watch someone sleeping, you will notice how their chest rises and falls in a rhythmic way; their shoulders are relaxed and their breathing comes easily and naturally in a deep, smooth and calming rhythm. Now consider your breathing at this moment in time. Is it similar to that deep, calm and natural rhythm or is it shallow and irregular? Does your breath feel shaky or fast-paced? Is your chest tight?

Although breathing is a natural and automatic process, by paying attention to it, you will find that you may not be breathing as effectively as you could be. By noticing your breathing and focusing on it during the practices and at other times, you can increase the levels of oxygen entering your blood stream and your brain, reduce your stress levels and the release of stress hormones, as well as promote your own sense of well-being. You will be building your internal resilience and resourcefulness, and gaining more awareness of why you respond as you do and how you can have control over your reactions and responses to what you feel, think and do, and the choices that you make.

Mindful awareness

The practice that follows is a cornerstone for mindfulness meditation. In this practice, the focus is on breathing into the core of your body, hypothetically into the area of your belly button. Developing a positive relationship with this practice, whether it be for 20 minutes or just for five minutes, can bring many benefits. It can help create or further develop a stable and connected anchor that you can focus on and hold on to in times of distress as well as when you are simply wanting to reconnect to that nurturing and balanced part of yourself. Along the harsh, uncertain and bumpy road of cancer, having something positive and gentle to anchor to is of enormous benefit.

There is no need to force anything or to feel pressurized. Emotions will be evoked and if they are then step away. Stop doing the practice or shift your thoughts back to your breathing. There is no need to force yourself if something feels uneasy, unpleasant or unhelpful. What is offered in this book has the sole purpose of providing you with an opportunity to try something new or different and to reinforce what you are already doing. It is a helping hand, but if it's not what you want or need right now, leave it. Put it aside, knowing that you can revisit it at a later stage should you so wish.

Meditation or sitting positions

You may find it more comfortable to sit upright in a chair, on your bed or cross-legged on the sofa. If you can't sit, then lie down, stand or find a position that suits your situation. Some people find sitting on a meditation cushion helps them to focus. These are large, firm, round cushions called zafus which help keep you upright. It is important whenever you are sitting for any period of time to make sure that the level of your hips is higher than your knees, even when sitting in a chair. There is no need for you to suffer, so use cushions, blankets or anything else to help you feel comfortable. Always try to keep your back upright and sit so that your chest and heart are open with your head gently balanced on your neck. There should be a softness and openness to your approach to all the practices.

There will always be noise but try and find a place where you won't be interrupted and ensure that your mobile is turned down. These meditations can be done sitting at an office desk, in a chair at home or on a bench in the garden. Some people find them useful to use during treatment or when waiting for a procedure.

No right way or wrong way

When doing these practices, there is no set way or special position you need to adopt. What helps is knowing that your mind will drift whenever you do a practice and that your thoughts will suddenly take on great importance now that you're trying to let them pass on. Minds drift and float; they think and produce pictures, thoughts, ideas, sensations and many other things – and that's because they are doing exactly what they are meant to do. Trying to stop this happening is pointless. What you want is to be aware of how these thoughts come to mind, what they are and how you can manage them. Acknowledge whatever is there without reacting, simply saying *thought* when a thought comes up or *feeling* when a feeling emerges. It's about recognizing the activity for what it is (e.g. thinking) and then letting it be there without attending to it.

When your concentration moves from your breathing, or when you find yourself getting into a conversation with yourself or someone else in your head about a topic, recognize this activity, step away from it and bring your attention back to your breathing – focus and refocus no matter how often this happens. This will happen repeatedly because your mind and brain are doing what they are meant to do. Your task is to manage and navigate your thoughts and responses and it is this management of them that will help to make such a difference to your life. Training yourself to recognize, acknowledge and let pass difficult, repetitive and unwarranted thoughts, self-criticism and judgement will not only provide relief but reset your attitude and brain pathways so that you can open up your life to kindness and balance. You won't need to go down each dark alley in your mind because, with practice, you will be able to stop, recognize what you're doing and reset your path onto something far more helpful and nourishing.

It cannot be stressed enough how essential it is that you keep doing the practices, as each time you do, you are developing the structures in your brain, your emotional resilience and your own internal sense of stability and belief. You will see that this encouragement recurs throughout the book as it is so important.

The following practice is one that you will come to rely on for years to come. It is one of the key meditations that is central to mindfulness practice and its benefits are far-reaching. It truly is worth doing on a regular basis, even if only for five or ten minutes a day.

Mindfulness Practice: Mindful Awareness

Mindful awareness is about becoming aware of what is happening within yourself which encourages you to bring your focus and attention to your internal experiences and how they shift.

🔊 There are two options for this practice on the audio download: a 20-minute version (entitled 'Mindful Awareness') and a five-minute version (entitled 'Mindful Breathing'). Begin with the five-minute version. When this feels familiar you can move on to the 20-minute one. Ideally, do the 20-minute version a few times per week, and the five-minute one on the other days.

Transcript of mindful awareness practice (five-minute version)

With your eyes closed, being alert and awake, bring your attention to your breathing, and to the movement of the breath as it comes in and out of your body. Simply observe your breathing – watching the path it takes as it travels in at the nose, down to the abdomen and then out again though the nose.

Staying focused on the breath, without forcing it in any way. Being here, with each inbreath and with each outbreath, letting one follow on from the other.

Use your breath as an anchor. Allow the breath to anchor you to the centre within your abdomen, that part that is stable, focused and present. Follow the breath to your anchor, bringing with it a new beginning and with each outbreath a letting go.

Be aware of each breath nourishing and grounding you, renewing and letting go, one breath following the other. Allow it to bring with it a stillness and a feeling of balance, grounding you right here, right now. Letting it anchor you, gently and kindly, to this moment, and to this moment.

As the intensity begins to ease, let your attention spread to include all of your body, and engage your breath into a rhythmic flow that moves in and out of your body as a whole.

Gradually let your awareness begin to take in the sounds around you and within you simply letting them exist in harmony with you, as you breathe. Sitting in stillness, in this moment.

Feeling grounded, feeling balanced. Gently allow all of your senses to be awake, to be alert and alive to all that is happening within you and around you. Acknowledge with kindness that you spent this time living each moment of your life, with whatever came with it, in a mindful, balanced and open way, and that you now have the choice of how you wish to live this moment of your life, and this moment.

9

First the shock, then the aftermath

During treatment, and once it has been completed, you may feel exhausted, constantly preoccupied with the cancer returning, guilty you survived while others didn't or struggle to adjust to your situation as it now is. Any of the following issues may come to the fore, such as:

- Suppressed or repressed feelings
- Relationship issues with a partner, family, friends, children, work, work colleagues
- New relationship issues, such as anger or resentment at a partner's behaviour, loss of interest in a partner, wanting more from a partner in general
- Changes in your view on life
- Things that have not been said in order to protect you or someone else that are now a problem
- Anxiety and fear that the cancer will return
- Physical complications or a new disability
- Post-treatment fatigue
- Sexual issues such as a new fear or dislike of sex, a disinterest in sex or sexual contact
- Complications from the illness and treatment
- Financial worries
- Enormous lifestyle changes
- Reduced quality of life – due to fatigue, money problems or permanent physical changes have come about
- Personality changes resulting from hormone fluctuations, medications or surgery.

Life is never the same after having cancer. Why should it be? It's never the same after any experience, even good ones. You can't go back to a time in the past – before children, before a relationship, before an illness or accident, before finishing school or university, before someone died. We can't travel backwards in time, nor can we time travel to the future. Life is what you have now, for all that has been.

There is a misconception that the all clear or being in remission will mean you no longer worry and that you can return to your old life and your normal way of doing things. You can't. You have changed physically and psychologically, and so has the life around you. Time has moved and with it came your experience, and that experience affected both you and others around you.

It can feel lonelier at the end of treatment than at the beginning when you were first diagnosed and everything kicked in. When you are diagnosed there is a good deal of support from professionals, friends and family. Now that has passed, people are getting on with their lives, your professional team have waved you goodbye – now what? Even close friends don't want to keep hearing about your fears or anxieties, not because they don't love and care about you, but because they too want to move on with life in a more hopeful way or feel they need to recuperate by not always talking or thinking about your illness or their own fears and concerns.

Recovery after treatment

- 'I ought to feel fine, happy and wonderful. Why don't I?'
- 'Why do I feel so fearful, exhausted and overwhelmed even though my treatment is complete?'
- 'I'm not ungrateful for being in remission but I feel awful and more fearful than before.'

These are common concerns after treatment. In addition, your attitude towards work, life and other people may have changed and that too can feel disconcerting. Your body and mind have been through hell and the trauma may be ongoing due to side effects, surgery, pain, medications and more. These ongoing effects could include a stoma, stents, nerve damage, scars, incontinence, loss of an organ or limb, disfigurement, a disability such as poor speech or inability to walk. On occasions, especially if there has been brain surgery, there can be personality changes such as an increase in aggression, depression, psychotic thoughts, irritability, fearfulness etc. Personality changes can also come about from medication such as hormone treatment or from the actual experience of having cancer.

Self-doubt can easily creep in about who you are now: whether you are as able as you were before this difficult experience; whether you are still lovable, capable or still enjoy the things you used to. There can be self-hate, body loathing. shame about your body or its functioning, and shame about how you feel. If you have undergone a mastectomy or need to wear a bag, or have experienced any other physical change, you may find that your body image is different now and you may struggle with it. Having scars, being incontinent, wearing pads or bags, losing a breast or limb all bring about big shifts in your perception of yourself. This may lead to not wanting physical closeness with a partner, now or in the future, rejecting sex or even touch, whether intimate or friendly. For some people, they may feel a sense of loss or incompleteness if they have had a limb or organ removed. What is worth noting is that getting into remission and the relief and pleasure of that doesn't mean that you won't have any difficult feelings or negative reactions.

Your eating habits may have changed through the loss of taste or appetite, a required change in diet or because of ongoing nausea, vomiting, flatulence or bowel movements. You may feel exhausted, resentful, disgusted, isolated, alone, in pain, depressed or constantly anxious. Your physical symptoms or side effects may last for months, years or never change, especially if there has been nerve damage, loss of a body part, brain damage or a body function such as sight or the ability to get an erection.

What is important to hold on to is perspective because illness and events can alter our perception of who we are. This change in perception is real but it can also become distorted. For example, the way you see things may not be the way others see them. You may feel disgusting and ugly, scrawny and disfigured, but that's not how others view you or your situation. The way we feel inside is transferred to others as though they feel the way we do. They often don't, so take care not to increase your distress by assuming others feel or see what you do.

A great deal of disharmony comes about from having expectations. You may have expectations of yourself and of others that are different from the reality of what you are able to do or what others may want of you. This can lead to anger, mistrust and confusion, so getting some awareness of both your expectations and those of others can help to clear the way for moving forward.

Keep in mind that negative feelings won't increase your risk of cancer, but stress will, and the more you put pressure on yourself and bottle up whatever is going on inside of you, the more likelihood there is of you becoming stressed.

You need time to readjust, to grieve for the loss of what you had or may never have again. It's important to sift through the harshness of your experience and the changes that have happened whether physical, psychological, financial, within your relationships or regarding work.

Mindfulness Practice: Mountain Meditation

🔊 The Mountain Meditation is designed to create a sense of stability, balance and well-being. It is about claiming this moment and this space for yourself, and anchoring yourself, no matter how distressing life may be. It is a reminder of your personal resilience, reassuring you that you can weather any storm, even in the face of pain. If you can't stand for this practice, sit in a chair or prop yourself up in bed.

Listen to the Mountain Meditation track. Once you have completed this, think about how you face difficulties, the storms you have weathered and the times that you thought you could not cope or that life was not going to get better. Hold in your mind what you think helped you to get through it.

Below is a transcript of the Mountain Meditation practice which you can find on the audio download.

Transcript of the Mountain Meditation practice

Stand with your feet hip-width apart so that you can balance yourself. Keep your knees soft and your hips loose, imagining there is a small weight attached to your tailbone (coccyx). Tuck your navel in towards your spine as though you are pulling in your stomach to tighten your belt. Relax your shoulders into your back, lightly tuck in your chin, and let your head balance on top of your spin. Breathe in, and on an out-breath let unwanted tension be released. On an inbreath take in a feeling of relaxed strength.

As you stand, be aware of your breath moving in at the nostrils, down the back of the throat, into the chest and down into the abdomen, and then its movement from the abdomen, through the chest and throat, and out through the nose. Allow a natural rhythm of breathing; not forcing the breath in or out in any way.

Whilst standing here, feel the weight of your body in your feet, firm against the earth and that the earth can carry your weight with confidence. Let your breath feel as if it is moving all the way down into your feet giving them strength and stability. Now let the breath move into your ankles, strengthening them, and now into the calves. Let it flow into your knees, without locking them, and then into your thighs. Move the breath and steadiness into your hips, genitals, buttocks and abdomen, and let this area of your body feel strong but relaxed.

Allow the breath and strength to move up your spine at the back, through your stomach and chest, eventually reaching your shoulders, checking that they are relaxed. Your arms becoming stronger and part of the mountain, stabilising you, balancing you. Let it move into your neck and jaw, into the skull, ears, face, eyes and right up to the top of your head.

Now, in your mind's eye, move the breath to the base of your spine and thread it like a piece of string through each vertebra from the tailbone, up through the pelvis, the lower back, the middle of your back, the shoulder blade area, the back of the neck and all the way to the top of your head where it exits and is held gently but firmly on a hook, allowing your body to hold itself.

Feel the sensation of this, of your body standing like a mountain, fixed and firm, gracious and solid. The mountain is stable and grand: the earth beneath it, the sky and air around it. The weather changes, the seasons move from one to another but the mountain remains. Feel the strength of the earth beneath you, solid and powerful, and your body open and alert, as you stand grounded and dignified in this space.

No matter how chaotic life may seem at times, you already have coping skills that you use on a daily basis as well as in stressful situations. Now you can build and develop even more resilience. Find that one thing within yourself, no matter how small, that you know is strong and firm and remind yourself of it each day.

Thoughts, emotions and experiences are transient, but the core of you is constant and enduring. By engaging in practices such as the Mountain Meditation, you are reinforcing your capacity to choose wellness over distress. Mindfulness is as much about celebrating your achievements, success and health as it is about negotiating the more difficult or negative experiences of your life.

Focusing on the present moment can increase your understanding of what has happened in the past and improve your chances of a calmer, more grounded future.

Cancer and your identity

When you have cancer there is often good support and strong connections are made. There are others who know your concerns and can identify with what you are experiencing. However, the downside of this is that the cancer becomes the focus rather than you, so take care not to lose your identity to the illness. Hold on to and remind yourself of your own individual identity. There is such a high incidence of cancer that it becomes quite easy to feel like you belong to The Cancer Club. Throughout the whole process of diagnosis and treatment, and through the issues that occur during and as a result of having cancer, it is easy to lose perspective and to over-identify with the illness (consciously or unconsciously) at the cost of forgetting that you are first and foremost you, a person, the person you were before the illness and still are, albeit with new experiences to add to who you are. An illness such as cancer, with all that comes with it from the start, can insidiously take over or overshadow your previous sense of self and identity. Take steps to remind yourself that you are still you, a man or woman, a friend, a mother, a father, a daughter, a carer, a professional and also a person with cancer.

There is a tendency to shift identity, your sense of self, from you to the condition. It becomes a label – 'I'm a cancer patient', 'I'm a mental health patient', 'I'm an alcoholic', 'I'm disabled' – as though that is the person. It's not. The condition isn't your identity – it is part of your identity but there is a big difference. In essence, don't lose your identity to a condition as the condition isn't all of you. It may have a profound impact on you, on what you can or can't do, or how you see yourself, but you are more than the condition. The condition doesn't have an individual, living set of experiences and a history of events from birth. Separate yourself from the condition, no matter how consuming it is in your life.

Mindfulness can help you to step away from yourself and to notice how you view yourself both as an individual and as part of the world now that you have an illness. Observe your response to yourself and your illness and know that you can take a meta view of both. Observe and notice your situation from above. This can help you to keep perspective and to hold onto your idiosyncratic identity.

A moment of thought

After a few weeks of doing the practices, think about what it was like when you first started doing them or even to the time before you started. Have you made a real effort or do you skip over the practices, only reading them or about them? Make a mental note or use a journal to make notes to see if you have noticed any positive or negative effects of the practices. Do you feel that you have been managing stressful situations differently since you have started exploring mindfulness work? What has motivated you to continue? If you have been doing the practices, what made you do them and how do you keep them going?

If you haven't, think about why not. You may find that there are similarities between this and how you generally approach new or difficult things in your life. Now is the time that you can either use the motivation that you have to keep going or address the disinterest or procrastination that has prevented you from moving forward with it, providing it's something you want to do.

The idea behind the approach in this book is to help you develop awareness of yourself and to encourage you to increase your resilience and belief that you are the one person who can make the most difference in your life.

10

Life and the prospect of dying

Dying is the process of getting to the end. Death is the end of life as we know it. Different cultures have different ways of dealing with death, dying and living. Within each culture are vast individual and familial norms and attitudes towards both being alive and dying.

What is your view of death, of others dying and of your own inevitable dying? You have cancer, but you may not die from it now or even in the future. Your cancer might never return. You might get cancer of a different form or in a different part of your body. If this happens, you can use what you have learned and experienced to face it again or to face any other challenge.

When the prospect of your own mortality slaps you in the face it's hard to find equanimity. Pain, loss, illness and death are inevitable, but suffering is only one option when life is harsh. Perhaps there is a gentler route that you can also consider, which will be discussed further on.

Loss

A sense of loss is something we experience on a regular basis, mostly in small ways, but sometimes in a more profound manner. Having cancer can bring about a loss of not only life but of lifestyle, work, confidence and many other things. What is often overlooked is the severity of the loss that can come through the illness, the treatment or the outcome. Major concerns include infertility, impotence, cognitive and memory difficulties, loss of quality of life, loss of income or status, or a loss of a sense of who you are. It also depends on the age at which you get cancer. If you are a young person you may feel that your life has been put on hold and that you are being left behind and missing out while your peers are off studying or living life, making plans and getting involved with projects and plans.

This does not only affect young people. If you have established your career or started a family, you too may feel different from your peers if you no longer have an interest in what you used to enjoy, are too tired to join in family or school events, or are too exhausted to excel as you once did. Losing a career and the financial stability it brought is often underestimated and is viewed as secondary to you responding well to treatment or now being in remission. However, this can change not only your financial status but your ability to pursue what you once loved or thrived on. You might lose the ability to engage in activities that once allowed you to feel connected and part of a community. Your mood may have dropped considerably over this difficult time, leaving you feeling depressed or anxious. Surgery may have left ongoing damage or distress that impinges on your ability to go out, walk, sleep, eat or be as you were before. The medications may influence how you feel and have unpleasant side effects or leave you with a long-term condition.

So much change and the feelings of loss are an additional issue you need to deal with. There are not only the physical effects but emotional and psychological ones too which can be more difficult to pinpoint or manage. You know that things change in life, but the difficult part is dealing with the ongoing sense of loss that comes with these changes and the enormous grief that can come from it, the sadness and pain of no longer having what you had in a significant area of your life. Loneliness and isolation are closely linked to no longer being able to socialize or take part in your favourite hobby or sport. Such activities are important and the damage caused by no longer being able to participate can lead to a deterioration in mental health. For those who are retired and, for example, play golf, losing out on the physical activity is one thing but what accompanies that is the loss of social conversations, events and engagement with your friends and peers. Your self-esteem and identity can be shaken, leaving behind a void as you don't always know what you now want to do or even if you can do it.

A further issue is that of fertility. This is a significant loss especially if you have been unable to have your eggs frozen. It's not only an issue for women but for men too as they may become temporarily or permanently infertile or suffer from impotence as a side effect of surgery or chemotherapy.

A significant area of loss that occurs is in your level of energy. Fatigue is a major factor resulting from chemotherapy, but others who have only had surgery may have it too. It interferes with so much and affects your quality of life as it's extremely difficult to engage in anything, even the basics of daily life, when you are so fatigued.

Other areas that can be affected by treatments are memory and cognitive functioning. Such difficulties can include struggling to find words, remembering things, thinking clearly, retaining information, keeping up in conversations and your head may feel fuzzy. These difficulties can occur during but also after chemotherapy and they can lead to frustration, embarrassment and communication problems.

Acceptance

Acceptance can often be misconstrued as something to which you acquiesce or agree to without resistance or when you give up the fight. Within the context of this book, its meaning is to do with knowing and being with your situation in a way that allows you to focus on what is good, present and real for now, rather than on what is wrong, missing and damaged.

Thich Nhat Hahn, a well-respected Buddhist, suggests smiling into our pain and sadness. It is a strange concept but one that can bring about a feeling of kindness and care to your distress. Focusing on what is, with the warmth and softness of a smile, rather than what is not, gives you the chance to be with your situation in a kinder way.

Resilience

You approach the obstacles and challenges in life according to your internal beliefs and experiences. At times you may find your resilience is not as you would expect from yourself or that it's less than you would like. The good thing is that you can learn to be resilient and mindfulness can help to increase the resilience you already have as it helps to give you a greater sense of stability in your life. You have most likely already been through hard times, so use what worked well for you then and build on it.

Resilience is like the internal structure of a building. You can't necessarily see it or even know how strong it is until it is put to the test. You can reinforce the parts that don't appear to be as strong and develop internal structures that may be missing or unsteady. This takes time as you need to learn and encourage a change in your responses and train yourself to come back to a better place within yourself rather than being swept away by powerful emotions.

The practices outlined in this book all contribute towards developing resilience in some way, by returning to the breath during a meditation, refocusing your attention on the soles of your feet or quietening your anxiety through counting while you breathe. Shifting your perspective will certainly help you to develop a greater sense of control which in turn will help when dealing with challenges. Remember that when things feel out of control you have the option of choosing how to deal with, react and respond to those feelings, thoughts and situations.

Engage with your life at every level and commit to living it as best you can for now, no judgement, no self-criticism. Know that you can influence your life by choosing how you approach it. One of the first steps is to be open to yourself about your responses and reactions. Even when things are denied they don't cease to exist; they just come out in a different way.

Recognize that things are different now, physically, emotionally and psychologically. You can't carry on with your life as if nothing has changed and all is as it was before the diagnosis and/or treatment. That was then, this is now, for whatever it is.

It is also helpful to be careful not to hold on to responsibilities in order to show others, or prove to yourself, that you can carry on as before, that nothing needs to change and that you can cope. Your life has shifted. Perhaps holding on is because of the fear that if you release your grip, you will fall apart, stop fighting, give up, get sicker or even die. Maybe you are scared you will scream, weep forever, crumble or shatter into pieces. These responses sound dramatic but they are real and the situation you are in will evoke very powerful emotions.

Pride often comes into play as does the image that you (and everyone else) present to the world: 'I'm fine', 'I can cope', 'I'm tough', 'I'm resourceful', 'if there's a problem I deal with it, I don't whinge and moan'. All of these can place a great deal of pressure on you when there is a life challenge like having cancer; it can't readily be managed and your resources may be feeling depleted. We fall into the trap of thinking that if we can keep the game face on then somehow we will get through intact.

No matter what you think, say, do or deny, you will still be you with an illness.

The fear of not knowing the outcome can be destructive and overwhelming. Draw it in and say, 'I'm here in this moment, that is all that I know'. Notice your breath, your breathing and being present. Ask yourself, 'Can I trust life enough to breath?'.

You may even think that if you exhale, if you ease up, then it means you are surrendering to your illness. You aren't; all you are doing is breathing in and breathing out in order to survive. Let yourself be held by your breath, by life and by all those who love and care for you.

Suffering

Harsh and difficult events affect your life just as pleasant and joyous ones do. A negative experience like having cancer becomes both physical and emotional. The emotional responses create suffering and it is frequently the suffering, the psychological and emotional distress that accompanies life situations and events, that increases your emotional pain. What mindfulness offers are the tools that develop your ability to step back and to shift the focus; it provides the opportunity to take back some control and to help ease your suffering.

First what is required is a willingness to create a different perspective on your illness and its consequences. It's about renegotiating your relationship with your condition and allowing a shift in attitude towards life to develop. By engaging in the practices, you are quietening your internal conversation and finding a deep quiet, a total presence within this moment. Meditation is about you, your life, your pain and your joy. It's far greater than a technique or exercise, although we talk of exercising our ability to focus, concentrate and be present in order to develop a mindful mindset or approach to life. Meditation does not seek a specific mental or meditative state; it's not something abstract, disjointed or separate. In fact, it's the very opposite – being present, engaged and active, moment to moment, is what we aim to develop and create. Doing the practices, the formal meditations, is where the work really starts as it is this plus the framework of a mindful attitude that allows you to establish and connect to that quiet strength and stability within yourself. It allows you to know that you have the option of approaching your distress in a way that possibly could bring about a sense of equanimity. There is a track entitled 'Gentle Space' on the audio download. This is a few minutes of quiet time, where there are no guided instructions but simple 'bong' sounds to remind you to come back to your breathing. As mentioned before, can you allow yourself to be quiet, to feel that gentle space of quiet? Can you turn towards your suffering so that you can, over time, turn from it?

By focusing on now, there isn't the space or time to think of the past or future. You can't ruminate or get into the things going around in your head – the stories, regrets, fears, angers and worries. Paying attention gives you a full experience of what is happening without thoughts of other things intruding. It opens you to thinking in clearer ways when you want to think, and your thinking becomes more coherent, specific and contained. You learn not to let your mind wander down dark alleys or into spirals that go into depression, fear and anxiety. Mindfulness teaches you, particularly through the practices, to label whatever is in your mind or body, such as a thought, a physical pain or a narrative, and let it drift on rather than stay with it and delve into it. The shadow of fear, whether of pain, loss or death, may be there, hanging over you with each breath. Let it be there but give yourself permission to also allow something else to co-exist with it, and what can co-exist is a sense of quiet, an anchor of peace or gentleness, or even acceptance.

Rest your awareness on the things that happen when you focus on your breath or on a task. Through mindfulness you are striving for a balanced internal state. However, balance is not all positive or all negative but a co-existence, a central point that can help you stand firm and realign during and after an intense or difficult experience, or even when something good happens.

We get blocked and stuck when there is difficulty or distress. Through meditation and focused breathing, you gently shift the block and tension around it and apply balance and care rather than a fixed negative focus on the source of the distress, i.e. your cancer. This helps you to unlatch from the suffering. The intensity of your situation may remain the same but there is less mental and emotional energy that goes into it so there is less suffering associated with it. Observing it with awareness and composure will allow you to see and feel the tiny changes that are happening moment to moment. By observing your distress with this intention, you get close up to the experience you are having but you then have the opportunity and skill to step back from it. When you step back, you give yourself the space to respond to your distress in a different way, to shift the emphasis and to take control of how you negotiate it. Do you go down the dark tunnel of choking fear or physical pain or do you recognize the difficult, often awful, situation but see it within a context where there is you, your situation and your response? Use your metacognitive capacity, both your metacognitive knowledge and metacognitive regulation to do this. Knowing that you have a choice regarding how you approach and respond to your cancer and suffering empowers you, but it will take work and time to develop this. The work will be in doing the practices, observing and noticing what happens, and allowing the unknown to become known to you.

Once you begin to do the practices, you will start to feel a great sense of relief, knowing that you can engage with and manage your distress through getting to know it, working with it and stepping back from it. Accept the situation, observe it and its variations, and allow a space between you and the cancer to be used by you in a way that is helpful and not destructive. By not rejecting or pushing aside the fact that you have cancer (nobody wants it but you have it), you can come to it with a gentle focus, an open observation of it and the process it takes, and then apply the care, kindness and compassion that you need.

When emotionally or physically distressed, you may feel ashamed, weak, pathetic, damned, angry, hopeless or a range of other things. By using mindfulness and compassion for it, you can ride the waves of distress that emerge and come out without feeling hopeless and damned. This also applies to those around you who see you so distressed. Get to know your distress, its shades and variations, its locations, degrees, durations and effects, how it ebbs and flows, if it shifts, what triggers it, what helps to ease it. Watch it and observe it with kindness and with a sense of gentle curiosity.

Resisting your emotional pain worsens it. The fear, judgement and anger build up in your mind and tension is created all over your body and sets off the stress response. You can't help resisting the distress as it's a natural and automatic response to something that is unpleasant and terrifying. You are geared towards survival, so you look to avoid what is unpleasant, but this avoidance isn't always in your best interest. The greater the resistance the greater the suffering as it increases your level of distress.

Plant a Seed of Quiet and allow it to grow.

- Feed it.
- Water it.
- Nurture it.
- Watch it.
- Take care of it.
- Cherish it, for it allows you to be with the preciousness of having this moment.

To summarize, the benefit of mindfulness is that it lessens your resistance, which in turn can help you to decrease your suffering. You can lessen your resistance in your mind and body through your attitude, observing your distress, doing the formal meditations and accepting that you are in some form of pain, emotional or physical. There will be distress at different points so meet it with kindness. Some may scoff at the idea of accepting your cancer or the distress around it, but acceptance is very different from surrender. Having cancer is frightening, the procedures can hurt and the fear is pervasive. It takes over your life but what you can do is work with it. Acceptance, as mentioned before, means awareness, stepping back from it and knowing it's there but not doing battle with it. Suffering distorts your perception, interactions and behaviours as well as uses up your psychological, physical and emotional energy. When you shift your energy from the fight you have more energy to do what is helpful and possible, maybe even more enjoyable, once the intensity subsides. Life is not static, nor are your emotions. You can develop and create a greater sense of equanimity around your situation no matter how despairing or heartbreaking it is.

Mindfulness will give you a new way of navigating your life through cancer.

11

Self-care

The idea of self-care is now a common feature in articles and resource material. Later in this book various topics around self-care in general are covered, but within this chapter the emphasis is on self-care within the context of mindfulness and meditation.

We know that caring for ourselves is important, especially when our minds or bodies are distressed. However, when it comes to feeding that part of ourselves that is within the emotional and soulful arena, we seem to find this more alien and particularly difficult to address or engage with in an ongoing manner.

The self-care meditation here is a gentle and nurturing one that aims to be simple in content. The focus is on reinforcing something good and kind that feeds you, rather than on a complex set of affirmations to instil in your mind. As with many things, it is the very simplicity of the self-care or compassion meditation that can make it even more difficult to do as it can evoke an emotional response. You may want to reject the nurture and compassion that you give to yourself because you don't believe you deserve it or feel that you are unworthy of receiving such kindness and love from yourself. Should you have a reaction to this meditation that is uneasy, stay with it and keep at it. However, don't push yourself in an unhelpful way but keep coming back to it and observe your response. Gradually give yourself permission to receive the compassion of the words and let it be held inside of you. Everyone is deserving of love and kindness. You can change the wording to suit your own ideas of generosity, kindness and care towards yourself.

Mindfulness Practice: Self-care and Compassion Meditation

This meditation is a starting point for developing a kind and caring attitude towards yourself. Sit quietly in any position that is comfortable for you and take a few gentle breaths. Repeat the following phrases to yourself.

- May I be happy and healthy.

- May I be safe and protected.

- May I live my life with ease.

Repeat these phrases over and over, even when it feels difficult. Simply notice and observe. There is no need to do anything other than breathe. Never push it, but allow whatever it is to unfold into your awareness, without judgement and only with kindness and compassion. Amid the chaos, you can find stillness and quiet for a moment, or a few moments.

Meditation can help with the wanting, holding on tight or too tight, seeking, clinging, fighting and battling. Surrender to the experience of the moment; surrender to what is true without judgement. Being non-judgemental means not placing a value or opinion on something, and more importantly, on yourself.

Be honest about what is happening. Mindfulness can help you to see, feel and be with whatever is present and happening. Not that you don't already know what is happening, but it helps you to be present with it in a different way. This may sound strange, but you will notice that you can bring something kinder to yourself through mindfulness.

It's about choice. What do you choose for yourself?

It is only natural that you will want to put more emphasis on pleasant rather than unpleasant experiences, but the harsh ones also need attention in order to manage them and recognize the impact they are having on your life. Mindfulness helps to influence how you react and interpret them. It can help you sustain your concentration and harness your internal resilience and resourcefulness.

Simply meet your experiences rather than react to them; don't let them push and pull you in different directions, causing you more conflict and pain. The practices are beneficial even if you don't like, believe or want to take on the philosophy and mindset of mindfulness.

Just like life, our brains aren't static. They can learn, create new ideas and concepts, new ways of thinking and being which is why mindfulness can be so powerful. However, it takes time and commitment. It can't help if you don't do any of the practices or engage with the concepts. Through using them you will start to think about what you are noticing now rather than where does this feeling or sensation come from.

You can use meditation to let your awareness unfold on a topic, theme or difficulty, for example, if you are feeling angry, worried about a procedure, fearful or exhausted. Go into it – don't avoid it. That's easy to say but you will get to know your limits and when you are at a point that is too much for now, leave it, come out of meditation or refocus your attention on something else. There is no need to tough it out or increase your distress. Meditation is there to help, not hinder or make things worse. However, emotions do arise in times of quiet so be aware and manage them.

Laughter and humanness

With the seriousness of being ill, it is hard to remember to laugh and to use humour. We are human and with that comes a capacity to not only suffer but to enjoy life.

There are good physiological reasons to laugh. It helps trigger endorphins, the same hormones that are triggered when we exercise. These are some of the hormones that can help us to feel good. Another is oxytocin which is released when we cuddle or hug, helping us to feel loved and warm inside. Laughter stimulates the immune and lymphatic systems, improves your circulation, reduces pain and muscle tension and helps to lower blood pressure.[1]

We so often forget to laugh, sometimes because we think it's inappropriate in such serious times or because we are simply too busy and focused on all the things to do in the day. Most children laugh a great deal and find many things hugely funny even if adults don't agree. As we get older, we put constraints on laughing, thinking we are mature and sensible by being more serious or that it is intellectual wit and clever comments that now count. Rekindle the enjoyment and sheer joy of laughing, just like children do.

Use humour to negotiate your struggle – instead of hating yourself for thinking or doing what you feel you shouldn't, laugh at yourself. Be human without being judgemental all the time; soften your attitude towards your humanness and your vulnerability.

Smile at yourself and smile at others because you are here for now, in all its awfulness, grace and glory.

Taking care of the carer

This section is written for a partner or carer, even for a family member or close friend.

As someone who is in a position of caring for a loved one with cancer, it is important that you also recognize your own needs despite what your partner, parent, friend or child is going through. Know that you can't change things for that person even if you are staring at him or her every second of the day and tending to every need. They will still be in pain, be fearful and anxious, be unable to sleep, be angry or irritable. They will still smile, laugh or be annoying. You are making an enormous difference, but it mustn't be at the cost of your health or emotional well-being. There is always the feeling that the person who is ill is in a worse position than you are, and that is most likely true, but perspective and balance also need to play a role and be part of your caring.

One essential factor is that you, as a carer, keep to some routine for yourself. This allows you to take care of some of your own needs, such as eating and getting exercise, going to the doctor or an appointment when required and getting a decent night's sleep, as it helps to keep a boundary around your role and allows you to attend to your life as well.

If you are a partner, you may have had to move into a separate bedroom. If so, try to keep that within a very specific timeframe. It is all too easy to adapt to being separated at night from each other. When no longer sharing a bed, it is even more important to keep the intimacy alive in whatever form possible. If you can't sleep together or have sex, cuddle in the evenings on the sofa, hold hands, shower together or chat outside after dinner or while it's cooking. Have a drink together (it doesn't need to be alcoholic) as that is often a good time to catch up.

As a carer or partner, it is essential that you both, or your family as a whole, find a suitable way to ensure there is some time together that is close, fun and warm, even if it is only for a short period of time every few days. The list of things to do and interferences from outside sources will always be there but making a space to enjoy each other's company is vital.

Don't be afraid to talk about your fears, concerns, needs, disappointments and stressors. By the same token, let the person for whom you are caring be allowed to express his or her concerns. There may be little either of you can do to change this but at least talking to each other about your situations and concerns helps both of you feel connected. One of the many obstacles encountered when someone has cancer is that others don't want to burden the person who is ill with discussions regarding mundane, everyday matters, but that is often what the person wants to hear about. Only talking about illness, treatments, side effects and an unknown future weighs heavy on everyone.

Your role is such a difficult one, but it is easy to get trapped in only giving and believing that you no longer have the same rights as before. Being the well one shouldn't lead to you feeling guilty but, unconsciously, watching a loved one suffer when you're able to go out, work and socialize can leave you feeling uneasy and even ashamed if you do enjoy yourself while your partner or loved one is ill at home.

Don't stop your life. You're still a person and the cancer shouldn't become a barrier between the two of you or be something that forces you to deny your needs. You may react by saying, 'Well, that's fine in theory but the reality is so demanding, intrusive, stressful and all-consuming that there isn't any space or time left for me'. The demands, stress and all the other factors will always be there but amid that, it is vital for you to keep hold of your own identity and needs. Just like the person with cancer, you are alive now so what choices do you want to make?

Join in as much as you can. Exercise together, plan together, discuss your needs, not only those of the one who is ill. Cook together, do some mindfulness practices together, discuss the news together, do the crossword together, go for a walk together. Work at keeping the togetherness there and let your partner or other person know that both of you need to work at keeping the closeness and enjoyment alive.

Be part of this in all aspects. Do not believe you must keep things going, shoulder all of it and be stoic. You are both suffering, in different ways for different reasons. If you don't take care of yourself then you run the risk of becoming ill, either emotionally or physically, and that won't help. Just as it is also the responsibility of the person who has cancer to take care of themselves in whatever way they can, it is equally important that you as the carer take responsibility for your own care. Remember, your rights don't evaporate when you become a carer. You're still a person.

12

Memories, pain, sleep and exercise

The experience of going through cancer can lead to a recurrence of memories, some of which may have felt extremely distressing, even traumatic for some. Not all memories are negative; it may also evoke those that are good and nourishing. In addition, your illness may also bring pain or increased discomfort, poor sleep and difficulties in being mobile and exercising. As these issues are hard to deal with, there will be a discussion here on each.

You may once have had a sense of faith and equanimity that now feels challenged or shattered, and your previous take on life and sense of hope and determination now feel diminished. You wish you could go back to what was your normal life, but you struggle knowing that you can't move back in time and your life now is different in so many ways. What mindfulness may offer is a way of finding underneath all this distress and chaos a sense of calm, even if only for a moment at a time.

Difficult memories

Distressing memories of treatment, procedures, complications or disruptions may re-emerge over time. If they do, it is useful to deal with them in some way. Most memories like this are upsetting but not so distressing that they create stress and unsettle the person when they continually reoccur. Most are not accompanied by other sensations or symptoms associated with post-traumatic stress such as hypervigilance, nightmares, racing heart, flashbacks and so forth. Recognizing the difference between the two is important.

Procedures, surgery and interventions are words, but they can feel like an assault through their intrusiveness and the relentlessness of being assessed, treated, prodded, poked and questioned. Add to this chemotherapy which can have extremely unpleasant after effects or side effects: vomiting endlessly for days; ongoing diarrhoea that causes intense stomach pain and sensitivity; nerve damage or psychological distress in which the emotional scars are far more difficult to heal than the physical ones. What about the pain that people endure from the cancer, surgery or nerve damage? It can strip away all quality of life. Events, experiences as well as pain are all believed to have a memory.

In general, the brain pathways that developed or were reinforced at the time of the trauma remain and are easily reactivated when something associated with the trauma happens, such as a similar smell, touch or simple behaviour. These triggers can remain from early infancy until death and can emerge to a greater or lesser degree depending on how much of the experience has been processed. When a disruptive experience occurs, the normal processing of material is interfered with, so the input or stimulation doesn't go through the usual channels in the brain that would normally allow for the experience to be analysed, interpreted, a context given to it, and finally, for it to be put into storage as an accessible and formulated memory.

With very distressing situations, the material associated with the experience isn't sufficiently processed, particularly in the section where it is interpreted and meaning given to it before being stored in the memory (the hippocampus). Consequently, this unprocessed or insufficiently processed material is easily activated, especially when there are triggers that remind the person consciously, but mostly unconsciously, of the past event. Triggers can flip you into reliving the experience in a nanosecond. For example, walking into a waiting room, receiving a letter, going for a check-up, the smell of a hospital. Certain triggers can throw you into a flashback experience where the experience is relived as though it were happening all over again, or else it can set off powerful thoughts about the event that are then difficult to put aside and can set the person on a downward spiral and evoke physical pain.

Having cancer is your personal explosion, like an earthquake that has shaken your very foundation. There can be tremors, aftershocks and debris, and the aftermath can be long-lasting. It takes time to rebuild or build new structures. If your memories are so distressing and interfere with your psychological recovery, it is helpful to seek professional help.

Below is a lovely practice that can be used on an ongoing basis. It is a very grounding practice and it can help if you are experiencing upsetting memories or thoughts, or simply feeling a little off balance.

Mindfulness Practice: Soles of your Feet

This is an excellent practice that you can use at any time, such as when you are in a meeting, on a crowded train and starting to feel agitated. Use it if you find your anger creeping in or you are feeling unsure of yourself. You can also do it when waiting in a doctor's reception area or sitting at home in front of the television.

- Place your feet firmly but gently on the ground. Bring your attention to the bottom of your feet.
- Feel the sensation of your foot against your sock, your sock against the bottom of the shoe and your shoe touching the ground. If your feet are bare, then feel the sensation of your bare flesh on the ground.

- Focus all of your attention on the soles of your feet.

- In your mind's eye, imagine you are breathing in and out through the soles of your feet.

Feel each of your feet expanding and then softening with each breath.

Imagine a sense of weight coming into your feet and this weight is firm, strong and stabilizing.

Let this sensation ground you as you breathe in and out.

Bring your attention back to whatever is happening around you.

Pain

Pain is one of the most difficult components to deal with, during or after treatment. It can be acute or become chronic due to side effects, complications, surgery or from the cancer itself. A full discussion on pain management is included here as it is so distressing and disruptive, particularly if it is chronic. It can lead to an ongoing decrease in quality of life as well as mental health problems.

As a non-medical intervention, mindfulness has been actively researched to determine its use for managing pain and increasing the perceived quality of life of the individual. The outcomes have been very positive and it's now an accepted and recommended intervention by professional bodies for use in these areas.[1]

We often say we are hurting when we experience pain. Depending on the severity, we may also feel discomfort, anguish or even agony as a result. However, the threshold to experience and withstand pain appears to vary considerably between individuals with different characteristics. For example, research has revealed a higher incidence of chronic pain and sensitivity to pain in women.[2]

The Biopsychosocial Model of pain discussed earlier in the book offers an explanation for how we experience pain differently. To recap, it suggests that biological factors (e.g. genetics), psychological factors (e.g. personality traits) and social factors (e.g. family and peer support) can all have a significant effect on pain.[3] Consequently, by using interventions such as mindfulness to assist with managing pain and reducing the distress associated with it, pain is no longer solely the domain of the medical profession.

Mindfulness offers an opportunity to develop your self-capacity to manage your pain. Just as with your distress and emotional responses, over time it can give you a greater sense of control over your response to the physical sensations you experience as well as your emotional reaction to it. The same approach can be applied to your pain as a means of lowering the intensity of suffering around it. Two major studies[4, 5] have found that mindfulness:

- is more effective than opioid painkillers
- has significant and ongoing positive effects on pain for women with primary breast cancer
- shows significant positive results for those with chronic low-back pain when compared with usual care (as did cognitive behavioural therapy (CBT)).

Importantly, these effects were still found at six months and 12 months.

The physiology of pain

The medical perspective is that pain stems from sensations that are triggered in the body. It is understood that when our nerve endings are stimulated, they take action. When we are injured, pain receptors called nociceptors are activated and shoot off a response. This electrical signal travels through the nerve, on to the spinal cord and then to the brain. The process works at lightning speed and the signal is sent in fractions of a second. Upon arrival at the brain, pain is directed to several areas for interpretation and analysis. For example, parts of the cortex interpret the location of the pain and decide whether this is a new kind of pain you are experiencing or not, as your brain needs to make sense of the situation.

Signals are also sent to the emotional hub in the brain called the limbic system. This system dictates your emotional response to pain. For example, some people will become frustrated or even irate and others may cry. Associations are built over time between physical sensations you experience and emotions.

The Gateway Theory

The theory behind the Gateway Theory[6] (or Gate Control Theory) of pain is that, as mentioned above, a situation occurs that sends a message via nerve pathways to your central nervous system (CNS) situated along the spinal cord. These messages are then sent to the brain which analyses and interprets them. The brain sends messages back to the spinal cord and through the central nervous system to give its analysis. This is when you physically register the pain.

The points of contact where the message hits the spinal cord, and later when the brain sends a message back, contain what are regarded as gateways or ports. It is at these gateway points that it is believed that pain can be renegotiated so that it is lessened or removed. This theory also emphasizes that physical, psychological, emotional and cognitive factors can trigger or aggravate the pain you feel but also, when managed correctly and consistently, lessen or stop the pain.[7]

This has enormous implications for pain management, especially chronic pain management, as there are factors that open the gates and factors that close the gates. Factors that open the pain gates are typically stress, tension, emotional states such as anger and depression, too much focus or mental energy directed towards the pain (continually thinking or worrying about it), lack of activity which can lead to poor mobility, stiff joints and low levels of fitness. Factors that close the pain gateways are activities that encourage and foster relaxation, contentment and well-being, mental engagement in interests that make you feel involved and activities that distract you from the pain, exercise and activity to increase your fitness levels and help release your body's natural pain killers as well as develop and keep your muscle tone and joint mobility, medications (prescription or over-the-counter).[3, 4]

Reactions to pain

Reactions to pain can be wide-ranging depending upon the severity of the damage. It can be experienced for a short, intense period or it can be drawn out over many years. What is certain is that pain is far more than sensory and neural communications. It can be thought of as a complex mix of personality, emotions, culture, experience, physiological sensations and responses. We can be more vulnerable to pain depending on our genetic make-up, our socioeconomic status and the environment in which we live.

The reaction to pain is reliant on a number of factors as it isn't a linear, one-way system of cause and effect. Your previous life experiences, current mood and beliefs about your ability to cope with pain can all play a significant role in the pain process. We often respond to current pain in line with past experiences of it.

Pain and emotional memory

As mentioned, pain too is believed to have a memory. Certain things can trigger the memory of past painful experiences and this comes flooding back, even though you may not be aware of what triggered it. This trigger can activate old memories of pain and the events around it as though they were happening in the present time, leaving you feeling distressed and uneasy. This reliving of the experience can re-evoke the physical pain that is associated with the past memory.

Intensity control

The mind feels pain and processes it. It sifts through the memories you have of pain experiences in the past in order to find a solution to your current pain. Although this is done as a way of remedying your current pain, what it inadvertently does is activate your old memories. If your pain is chronic then a solution isn't found and you are left with re-evoked thoughts, emotions and memories of past pain. This can lead to feelings of distress, fear, anger or hopelessness which, in turn, increase your levels of stress and lead to a decline in physical and emotional health, a decrease in your immune system, an interruption to the healing process and a decrease in your quality of life.

This activation controls both the intensity and duration of the pain and your brain, through repeated cycles of pain, becomes more attuned and sensitive to pain as it now has more neuronal pathways developed in it that light up and activate whenever there is any pain or anticipation of pain.[1]

Mindfulness is now a well-established and verified intervention to help manage pain. You will find that the body focus meditation outlined earlier in this book is particularly helpful for pain, so you may wish to use it even if you have not taken to the other practices.

Sleep

Being ill triggers many thoughts that often seem to emerge in the quiet hours of the night. It is so easy to ruminate in those hours even though little is achieved from it. Mood changes can affect sleep, and depression and anxiety frequently interfere with restorative sleep. However, poor sleep can lead to low mood and poor functioning. A further difficulty is that you can sleep but still feel fatigued.

Treatments frequently interfere with sleep due to worry, pain or the effects of medications or surgery. Such interferences can be from nausea, frequent urination or bowel movements, joint pain, pain from surgery, constant thirst or physical discomfort. It can also trigger night sweats, menopausal symptoms and restlessness. Treatment interferes quite dramatically with your routine and it can inhibit physical activity.

There is one aspect of sleep that is widely recognized and that is our body's circadian rhythm. In essence, this refers to your internal 24-hour body clock situated in your hypothalamus. It goes in rotating cycles of wakefulness and tiredness throughout a 24-hour period, with each cycle lasting around 90 minutes during which you are more alert and then your energy levels dip. Once the dip has passed, you move up again into a more awake state. When asleep, during a cycle you go through different stages of sleep with the last being rapid eye movement (REM). The function of this stage of sleep is that it helps to form new memories, stimulate the central nervous system and the regions of the brain involved with learning as well as restore brain chemistry to a normal state. Equally important is the stage of deep sleep as it is essential for physical renewal, hormonal regulation and growth. Without this stage of sleep, you are more likely to get sick, feel depressed and even gain weight.

With these facts in mind, you can understand why establishing a good sleep pattern is so important. The key is to try and go to sleep when you are at the dip part of the cycle. That is the time to have your head on the pillow rather than fall asleep in front of the TV or decide to make a hot drink before bed. If you push through that window of tiredness the next opportunity will be about 90 minutes later. It helps to become familiar with your cycles. Try to notice what happens through the day, especially in the evenings, and at what times.

Adults need seven to eight hours of sleep a night. It is very tempting to sleep more than you need to when feeling fatigued or as a way of blocking out any low mood, anxiety or fearful thoughts. Sleeping during the day interferes with a good pattern of sleep at night. A quick nap of no more than 20 minutes during the day only is alright, but you should never do this in the late afternoon or close to bedtime.

Inevitably, stressors and anxieties of your situation and of the day are active but it is important to work with your body and to try and get some structure in place if you are to develop a healthy sleep pattern or curtail a disrupted one. Part of the problem if you are not getting enough sleep is that your head (emotionally and psychologically) doesn't get to have time out.

Keep a note of the following parts of your routine.

- Mealtimes
- Bath
- Time spent watching TV or using a computer
- When you go to sleep
- How often you wake up
- What you do when you wake up at night
- What time you wake up in the morning
- What time you get out of bed

A bedtime routine is essential for adults, just as it is for children. Rules to follow include:

- No computer
- No caffeine
- No sweets
- No rushing around
- Eating meals at a regular time
- Exercising at a regular time
- Having a bath at a regular time
- Going to bed at a regular time
- Preparing for sleep.

There are some other rules that are well worth sticking to in order to help your sleep pattern:

- Get out of bed if you can't sleep rather than toss and turn for hours. It is helpful to identify what is keeping you awake and to use self-talk to help you step away from your thoughts.
- Don't allow yourself to ruminate. Nothing is achieved except that you are not sleeping and you are depriving your body and mind of essential rest. Put your ruminations aside and give yourself permission to fall asleep or to at least be resting your body. Only allow yourself to ruminate in a different room, not in your bedroom. It can help to imagine putting your worries on the bedside table and telling yourself that you will come back to them in the morning; they will still be there.
- No chatting if you are awake and your partner is asleep – your partner is not to be woken up for a conversation.
- No eating or watching TV in bed. Sleep and sex are all that's allowed (or reading a book for a short time). No long

conversations, no smartphones or computers. These are absolutely off limits.

- Only watch TV in the lounge. Do not fall asleep there. It interferes with your circadian rhythm, so watch for when you generally start getting sleepy and work around it. Our sleepy times tend to come every 90 minutes or so.
- Have a bath, get into night clothes, brush your teeth, do whatever needs doing, including putting the bins out, putting the dishes in the dishwasher, locking the doors etc. Do all this before you sit down to relax.
- Go to bed before you fall asleep in front of the TV or when reading in the lounge. If you start to feel tired or sleepy then go straight to bed, turn off the lights and go to sleep. Don't start reading, checking your phone, making a list of things to do tomorrow. Go to sleep.
- Your phone must be off or turned over. Switch off alerts, email pings etc. Only keep your phone ringer on if it's essential.
- Make your room as dark as possible when you are trying to sleep. Be careful of all those little plug lights, radio time lights and other similar things as they too give off light.
- Try to avoid working in your bedroom.
- If you live in a small place, then separate the sleep part of the room and the work part with a divider or put your desk in the corner. There must be some differentiation.

Work with sleep problems and work around them. It takes effort to adjust to a healthy sleep pattern and environment and you may need a new arrangement during or after treatment.

- Get comfortable bedding, a new mattress if necessary, wear headphones if you or your partner need to listen to music or a mediation before falling asleep.

- Use separate bedding if you have a partner as it helps both of you if you are a restless sleeper or need different layers through the night. Some mattresses are available that reduce the bouncing effect of a partner when tossing or turning.
- Make sure your room is at a comfortable temperature, not too warm or too cold.
- If there are any items you are likely to need during the night, keep them close by, for example, a facecloth, a bowl of water if you want a cool cloth, dry pyjamas, a fan, a glass of water, some biscuits or a piece of fruit.
- Once you are well enough or in remission, change your room around and even look to redecorate it.
- Separate your sick bed from your sleeping bed by reframing the idea of bed, rest and sleep.
- See your bedroom as a good place, not a place of illness, fear and rumination.
- Try breathing and counting in a repetitive way – breathe in, 2, 3, 4; breathe out, 2, 3, 4. Do this repeatedly. If you start thinking about other things, simply come back to the exercise.

If you find you are falling asleep earlier than you expected or before your regular bedtime, it's alright to go to bed early but take care that it doesn't lead to you waking in the early hours of the morning and not being able to return to sleep.

People often seek out medication to assist with sleep, but it is not always the best route. There is frequently a rebound effect in that you may sleep the first week or two but once you stop taking the medication you find it extremely difficult to get to sleep on your own. Their efficacy lessens over time and they are mostly addictive.

It is helpful to keep in mind that If you have always been a poor sleeper then it's likely you will be one during and after treatment too. Like all things, it's about managing your sleep and problems that interfere with it, such as anxiety, pain, eating, hot flushes, irritability and so forth. Remember, mind, body and attitude all interconnect.

Exercise too is important for sleep quality, so keep as active as possible. The following section will focus on the benefits of exercise at different points of treatment as there is often a tendency to retreat from it when ill.

Exercise

Get some exercise. Unless you are bedbound it's important to try and expend the build-up of energy and frustration. Some people like to exercise early in the day, others later. It doesn't really matter what time you do it as long as you do it on a daily basis. It also releases endorphins which make you feel good.

The research on exercise before, during and after cancer treatment is positive. It should be noted that most of these studies were either undertaken with large numbers or involved an analysis of a pool of studies so the number of participants would be in the thousands or hundreds of thousands.

- In a study[8] of 1.44 million participants, it was found that leisure-time physical activity was associated with lower risks of many cancer types. Healthcare professionals counselling inactive adults should emphasize that most of these associations were evident regardless of body size or smoking history, supporting broad generalizability of the findings.
- Women who had a history of exercise activity had a 20 per cent lower risk of developing cancer, and this was found to be the same for both black and white women. This, however, was not the case for women who had a first-degree family history of breast cancer.[9]

- In an analysis of 20 studies, the findings confirmed the conclusions of other reports that the greater the levels of physical activity, the lower the risk of developing colon adenoma, and that physical activity may have an important role in colon cancer prevention.[10]
- It was found[11] that a six-month home-based, telephone-delivered exercise intervention of primarily brisk walking was associated with improved physical health-related quality of life (HRQOL) in women with ovarian cancer. HRQOL and exercise have both been associated with overall survival in women diagnosed with ovarian cancer.
- In a trial[12] 301 breast cancer patients took part in supervised exercise during chemotherapy three times a week. A higher volume of aerobic exercise (50 to 60 minutes) or combined aerobic and resistance exercise (50 to 60 minutes) was found to be both achievable and safe during breast cancer chemotherapy and this exercise might help to manage declines in physical functioning and worsening symptoms better than standard amounts of exercise, that is 25 to 30 minutes of aerobic exercise.
- Limiting weight gain during adult life, avoiding becoming overweight or obese, reduces the risk of post-menopausal breast cancer and cancers of the colon, endometrium, kidney (renal cell) and oesophagus (adenocarcinoma).[13] There was sufficient evidence for the role of physical activity in preventing colon and breast cancers, and limited evidence for prevention of cancers of the prostate and endometrium. Excess body weight and physical inactivity account for approximately one-quarter to one-third of cancers of the colon, breast, endometrium, kidney (renal cell) and oesophagus (adenocarcinoma). Thus, adiposity and physical inactivity appear to be the most important avoidable causes of these cancers.

- It was found[14] that physical activity was clearly associated with reduced risk of endometrial cancer, with active women having an approximately 30 per cent lower risk than inactive women. Regardless of the amount of exercise done, the more time spent sitting, the greater the endometrial cancer risk. In essence, the evidence now convincingly indicates that physical activity prevents or reduces risk of endometrial cancer.

- In a study[15] over 11.6 years with 8,034 invasive breast cancer cases, it was found that among women diagnosed with breast cancer after age 50, the largest risk reduction factor was found to be in those with the highest levels of physical activity. For cancers diagnosed before age 50, the strongest associations were found for moderate total physical activity. Household activity levels were also associated with lower levels of some types of tumours. The results of this, the largest prospective study on the protective effects of physical activity, indicate that moderate and high physical activity are associated with modest decreased breast cancer risk.

- Results suggest a decrease in risk associated with recent recreational physical activity, even of modest levels. The researchers also noted that starting or maintaining physical activity after menopause may be beneficial regarding breast cancer risk.[16]

- Physical activity could significantly reduce the risk of breast cancer with there being an increase in reduction associated with an increase in the amount of physical activity (i.e. the more exercise done, the lower the risk of developing breast cancer).[17]

- There appears to be an inverse association between physical activity and prostate cancer (PCa) risk, albeit a small one. Given that increasing physical activity has numerous other health benefits, men should be encouraged to increase their physical activity in both occupational and recreational time to improve their overall health and potentially decrease their risk of PCa.[18]

- There is some indication that leisure-time physical activity is associated with reduced risk of developing lung cancer among smokers.[19]

- A study[20] examined the strength, consistency, dose response and biological plausibility of an association between physical activity and risk of colon, breast, endometrium, lung, prostate, ovarian, gastric, rectal, pancreatic, bladder, testicular, kidney and haematological cancers. It also estimated the population attributable risk (PAR) for physical inactivity and cancer in 15 European countries. It found that there is strong and consistent evidence that physical activity reduces the risk of several of the major cancer sites, and that between nine and 19 per cent of cancer cases could be attributed to lack of sufficient physical activity in Europe. Public health recommendations for physical activity and cancer prevention generally suggest 30 to 60 minutes of moderate or vigorous intensity activity at least five days per week.

- Low and moderate intensity aerobic exercise programmes were significantly and equally effective in improving physiological and psychological function in a population of cancer survivors. Aerobic exercise appears to be a valuable and well-tolerated component of the cancer rehabilitation process.[21]

Whichever way you look at it, exercise is extremely important, but it should be graded according to fitness levels and approached in a realistic and responsible manner. Your body can't function well if it's not being moved around. Exercise also helps with stomach and bowel problems such as bloating and constipation which are common side effects of chemotherapy and medications. Fatigue is a well-known and often debilitating effect of treatment, so these suggestions are not provided lightly. However, both mindfulness practices and exercise are proven interventions to ease and manage fatigue.

It is difficult to get motivated, especially if you have never been inclined to exercise or if you are feeling tired and unwell. However, it is possible to become more motivated once you have made the effort – and there is no getting away from the fact that you will need to make an effort. Go walking with a group, friends, a walking club or borrow a dog. Get to the gym when it is quiet or join a Pilates or yoga class. Many people are embarrassed when starting something new but use your mindfulness practices to help you step aside from these feelings and engage in what is helpful and necessary for your well-being. You can be embarrassed or anxious but still do it. The one shouldn't preclude the other.

This is a time when you should also listen to your body so that you don't push yourself too far too quickly. That's the best way of dropping out and not resuming. Know when you are tired, or too unwell. Pace yourself and know that your emotions lodge in your body too so fear and anxiety might make you scared to continue when your heart beats quickly or you might be anxious that a stretch might pull on your scar even though you have been told you can go ahead and do it. Having said that, it is your responsibility to take care and to know when to stop. It's your body, inside and out.

13

Get moving

This section gives instructions on how to perform some gentle but useful moves to keep you flexible and to get you going. However, if you are unable to do any of them, there is an excellent mindful walking meditation that most people should be able to manage, even if only for a minute or two.

Most importantly, take care and be sensible. Don't do anything until you have been given the go ahead. If you have just had surgery or your scars haven't yet healed, extra care must be taken. If you feel dizzy or unsteady on your feet, hold onto the back of a chair or sit down. Alternatively, ask someone to be in the room with you. There will be more detail on this later.

Movement keeps your muscles and joints in better health and prevents the effects of further disruption caused by inactivity, such as poor circulation, muscle wasting, stiffness and so on. The effects are not only physical but psychological, as being cooped up and immobile can lead to isolation, depression and fear.

It is essential that you get moving. The only time you shouldn't is if you have specifically been advised not to.

The benefits of regular activity include:[1]

- up to 35 per cent lower risk of coronary heart disease and stroke
- up to 50 per cent lower risk of type 2 diabetes
- up to 50 per cent lower risk of colon cancer
- up to 2 per cent lower risk of breast cancer
- 30 per cent lower risk of early death
- up to 83 per cent lower risk of osteoarthritis

- up to 68 per cent lower risk of hip fracture
- 30 per cent lower risk of falls among older adults
- up to 30 per cent lower risk of depression
- up to 30 per cent lower risk of dementia.

There are many things you can do to increase movement and activity levels in your life, even if you are stuck in a chair.

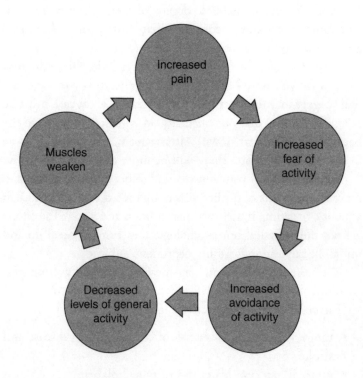

Mindful body movement

The following movements are gentle stretches to increase and maintain mobility. It might be that even these moves are not possible at the moment as you may be severely ill, bedridden, in too much pain or too frail. Should this be the case, other exercises can be done. The point is that whatever you do, no matter how small, it can be done in a way that integrates the movement with your breathing in a mindful and caring way. Seek advice if you are unsure of something and monitor yourself closely in order to prevent any injury.

These movements are only suggestions and are not a substitute for continuing with any other intervention you have been recommended. They can ease you into gentle activity if you have tended to shy away from it in the past.

> Key points to note:
> - It cannot be emphasized enough that you should only attempt what you can realistically manage.
> - If you have any physical difficulties have someone nearby who can assist you if needed.
> - Stand on a non-slip surface in bare feet or wear non-slip shoes.
> - Do not wear heels or socks if you are on a slippery surface.

It might be beneficial to do the moves with someone else. One person talks it through while the other does it and then switch around. That way both of you get to do it and can help each other. Many of the exercises can be done sitting in a chair, although this should be a chair without arms, such as a dining room chair.

Standing movements (or performed on a chair)

If standing, have your feet hip-width apart so that you can balance yourself. Keep your knees soft and your hips loose, imagining there is a small weight attached to your tailbone. Tuck your navel in towards your spine as though you are pulling in your stomach to tighten your belt. Relax your shoulders into your back, lightly tuck in your chin, and let your head balance on top of your spin. Breathe in, and on an outbreath let unwanted tension be released. On an inbreath take in a feeling of relaxed strength. This is referred to as the neutral position.

Be aware of each movement and let your breath flow in and out, without forcing it or breathing too deeply.

Shoulder shrugs

This can be done standing or sitting on a chair. If standing, be in the neutral position, let your arms hang loosely by your sides. Breathe out, lift the shoulders up towards the ears. Hold them there, breathe in, and as you breathe out, relax the shoulders down into the back. Repeat four times.

Shoulder circles forwards

The next move involves shoulder circles in a *forward* direction. From a neutral point, bring your right shoulder up to the ear, rotate it forward, down, around the back, and then towards the ear and continue with three more circles.

Repeat this move four times with the left shoulder, returning to the neutral position at the end.

Shoulder circles backwards

Now do *backward* shoulder circles. From the neutral position, lift your right shoulder up to your right ear, then rotate it back towards your shoulder blade, down towards the floor, forward and then up to the ear. Continue with three more circles, relaxing your shoulder at the end of it.

Repeat four times with the left shoulder, returning to the neutral position at the end.

Chest stretch

The first section of this can be done standing or alternatively sitting on a chair. Check your posture so that your feet are hip-width apart, your shoulders relaxed and your head gently balanced. Let your arms hang at your side.

This move is like a bird spreading its wings out to the side and then bringing them in again. So, with your arms down cross your hands in front of you. From this position, inhale while you extend both arms to shoulder height, arms parallel to the floor, and on an outbreath, bring the arms back down so that your hands cross over each other. Repeat this three times in a flowing movement.

Now, after spreading your arms out as described above, gently bend the knees at the same time as you bring your arms down to cross your hands. Then, as you lift your arms up again, straighten your knees. Repeat this three times at an easy pace and then relax your knees and arms.

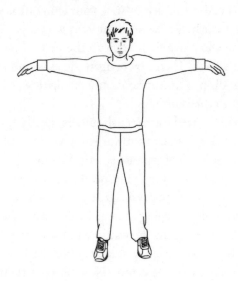

(a)

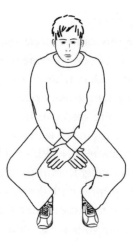

(b)

Neck and shoulder tension release

This can be done sitting or standing. Have relaxed but strong shoulders, i.e. don't slouch or stick your chin out as you can hurt your neck. Gently tilt the head forward so that your chin moves towards the chest and then lift it to the neutral position. Don't tilt the head back. Then slowly drop the chin and raise it again, and gently drop it and raise it, and finally lower the chin and come back to the centre.

Now with relaxed but erect shoulders, gently turn your head to the left, bring it back to towards the centre and then turn it to the right in one flowing movement. Without forcing it repeat three times and then bring your head back to the centre.

From the central position, gently tilt your left ear towards your left shoulder, keeping the ear in line with the shoulder so that your head isn't tilting forwards. Keep your shoulders relaxed. Only go as far as is comfortable and breathe into it (count to eight). Come back to the centre. Now tilt your right ear towards your right shoulder, keeping a straight line and not forcing it (count to eight). Return to the central position and repeat.

Now breathe out and slowly drop your head to your chest releasing any tension, breathe in and as you breathe out raise your head back to the neutral position. Repeat three times.

Full arm circles

The following movement is a full arm circle and can be done sitting or standing. Be careful not to breathe too deeply, but rather to allow the flow of breath to go with the movements.

Standing in a neutral position (or sitting), bring your hands to cross in front of you. Breathe in as you start to circle the arms around, with the arms crossing as though you are removing a jumper or T-shirt, and continue with the circle, breathing out as the arms come down. Breathe in and continue the circle upwards, breathe out as your arms come down. Repeat twice, then relax with the arms by your sides.

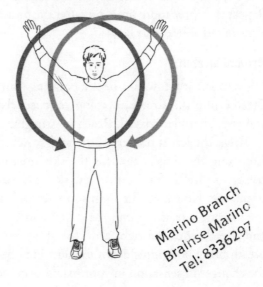

Arm lifts

The focus of this movement is on lifting the arms. Standing upright (or sitting), breathe out and lift the right arm up in front of you all the way until the back of your hand is up towards the ceiling, keeping the elbow soft and the arm rounded. Breathe in and bring the arm down towards your side. Repeat this three more times. Relax the arm, change to the left arm and repeat the movements.

Arm lifts alternating

This can be done sitting or standing. Both arms will now be used, but we will alternate them. Keeping the same posture as before, check that your hips are facing straight ahead if you are standing, and that your weight is evenly spread. Place your arms by your sides, and then lift your left arm towards the ceiling; as you bring it down lift the right arm up towards the ceiling, so that the arms cross over with the one arm following the other. Repeat this three more times but after the fourth time keep both arms raised above your head.

Upward stretch

Lift your left arm towards the sky, pointing your fingers upwards. Breathe into the stretch, keeping your feet flat on the ground and your shoulder relaxed. Reach up straight.

Relax the left shoulder a little and switch to the right arm, stretching the fingers towards the sky, reaching up as though trying to pick a cloud out of the sky, without tilting or over-stretching. Now relax the right shoulder and stretch again with the left one, breathing into the stretch, and relax that shoulder and stretch with the right arm, breathing into it. On an out-breath bring both arms down to your sides, becoming aware of the changes in sensation in your hands, arms and torso.

Side bends

The next movement involves gently bending sideways and can be done sitting or standing. If you are standing, relax your shoulders into your back, with your hips facing forwards, your feet apart, your knees soft. With your arms relaxed by your sides, breathe in and on an outbreath gently run your right arm down the side of your right thigh so that you are bending your body from the waist and allowing the left side of your body to be stretched. If you are doing the exercise in a sitting position, make sure your arm is straight and move your fingers towards the floor. Only go as far as you can with this movement. Watch that your body is in a straight line and that you aren't leaning forward or twisting your shoulders.

Breathe in, and on an outbreath come back to the upright position using the muscles in the core of your body to lift you and not just your shoulder. Check your posture, and on an outbreath bend to your right three more times, remembering to breathe and to bend from the waist in a straight line. Return to the centre.

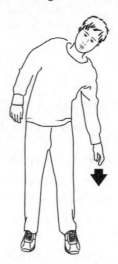

(a)

Repeat the same movement four times on your left side, remembering to breathe, and then return to the centre using your core muscles and bending and straightening up from the waist. Notice the areas of tension and when you tend to stop breathing. At the end, return to the centre position.

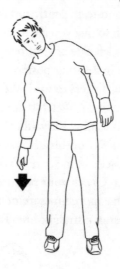

(b)

Floor movements

Now place yourself on the floor, if you can, as the following moves will be done lying on a mat or soft carpet.

Foot circles, foot flexes and one-leg circles

Lie on your back with your knees bent. Roll your hips slightly to ensure that they are evenly placed on the mat or carpet. Check that your spine is keeping its natural C-shaped curve in the small of the back. This is the relaxation position.

Bend the left leg towards the chest and clasp your hands behind the left knee – not on the knee but on the back of the thigh just below the knee – so that your calf is parallel to the floor. Gently circle the left foot clockwise four times, keeping the movement continuous.

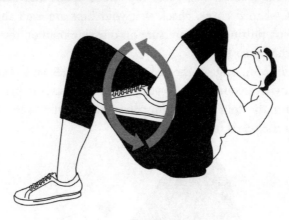

Now circle it anticlockwise four times.

Check that the upper part of your body is relaxed. Still holding your thigh, point the toes of the left foot towards your chin and then in the opposite direction away from you, repeating this four times. Remember to breathe naturally.

Now hug your left knee closer to your chest releasing the tension and return the foot to the floor.

Now repeat the whole set of moves with the opposite foot, i.e. using the right leg. Check that the upper part of your body is relaxed. Still holding your thigh, point the toes of the right foot towards your chin and then in the opposite direction, away from you. Again, repeat this four times, remembering to breathe naturally. Now hug your right knee closer to your chest, releasing the tension, and return the foot to the floor.

Extend both your legs out so that you are lying straight on the floor for the next exercise.

Pelvic tilt

We will now get the pelvis and lower back moving. So, lying on the floor, knees bent, feet hip-width apart, and the spine in its C-shaped curve, check that your hips are even and that you aren't putting more pressure on one side than on the other. Relax the upper body.

Breathe in, engage the pelvic floor muscles and pull your navel towards your spine. As you breathe out, start to press your waist into the floor so that your pelvic area begins to rise, slightly curling the pelvis inwards.

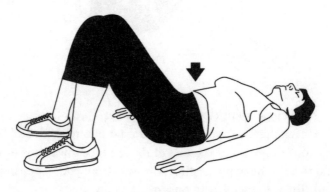

(a)

Keep your hips on the floor and hold this position. Breathe in, breathe out, breathe in, and on the next outbreath slowly roll the pelvis back to its neutral position.

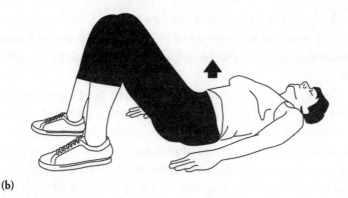

(b)

Ending off

Roll onto your side. Carefully and gradually bring yourself up from the floor, pausing for a moment before standing up. There is no rush and be cautious not to force or jar your body.

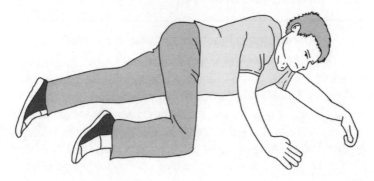

A complete set of movements can be found on the CDs accompanying the book *Life Happens* (www.lifehappens-mindfulness. com/books/life-happens/, also available as an MP3 download).

Try one or two moves and become familiar with them before moving onto the next one or two. This will help you to know which ones are manageable and which are too painful or difficult.

You don't need to be attending the gym or running around a field in order to keep fit. The gentle moves provided in this chapter can help to introduce you to greater body fitness or to restart it. They can also be used in conjunction with other exercises or even adapted to suit your situation. Whatever the case, taking care when exercising and breathing correctly when doing so is important for our health and safety.

A walk with a difference

The following is a formal mindful movement practice which is easy to do if you are able to walk.

Mindfulness Practice: Let's Go for a Walk

This practice is an example of an activity that you may do frequently without paying any attention to what you are doing. It has been adapted from the traditional walking meditation to include a broader perspective. Focusing your attention on to your automatic functions can ground and balance you, and this walking practice can be used when anxieties and stresses seem to be getting on top of you. Try it as a short break from work, studying or activities, or when you can feel your frustrations growing.

- Take a walk in the garden, a park or wherever is convenient. Keeping your eyes lowered, bring your attention to the physical sensations of walking. Feel the changes in pressure as you place your feet on the ground, be aware of your breathing, pay attention to the rhythm of your footsteps and the slight swinging motion of your arms. Acknowledge any emotions or sensations that come into your mind.

- Lift your eyes to the world around you. Little by little, pay special attention to the sights, sounds and smells of your environment. Take everything in: the movement, the stillness, the light, the shade, the chaos and the peace. Allow yourself to be open to your environment and its effect on you.

- Shift your focus to your connection to the outside world and the impact you are having on your environment. Let your breathing flow naturally, becoming part of the world around you. Feel the stability of the ground beneath your feet and let it strengthen you. Notice any changes in the sensations and feelings you are experiencing and acknowledge that the world around you is having an impact on you, just as you have an influence on the environment.

- Finally, take a mental step back from such an active involvement in the sensations of the environment. Continue to observe your breathing gently as a space forms between you and the outside world. You are aware of your surroundings, sensitive to them and appreciative of them, but the sensations arising from them are not the entirety of your experience. Take a moment to appreciate this moment, knowing you can take this sense of peace and clarity with you when you step back into your everyday activities.

14

Gratitude

Gratitude may seem a strange concept to raise within the context of illness and suffering, even the possibility of dying. Naturally, it's not about you being grateful for your condition but about keeping perspective so that you can still recognize the good that you have in your life. Gratitude can increase determination, attention, enthusiasm and energy[1,2] in adults and adolescents. For people with chronic pain it can help improve sleep and decrease depression; with improved sleep comes reduced anxiety.[3] Practising gratitude is strongly correlated with improved well-being.[4] Gracefully being aware of, and acknowledging, what you have in your life is a powerful antidote to distress.

Life isn't perfect and for many reading this book there are probably aspects of it that strip away at your very core. It is rare that you can find nothing in life to feel some sense of gratitude about, even when facing a terminal illness. Gratitude is about finding value in life and respecting that which is good, no matter how small – a smile, a warm bed, a kind friend. Gratitude helps you to be attuned to the nuances of life and to be thankful for those who bring you comfort, pleasure or greater understanding.

When you view your life through eyes that notice all of life, the good and the harsh, and you feel a sense of thankfulness for those aspects that are positive, loving and kind, no matter how small, it helps you to keep perspective. A smile from a stranger, laughter with a friend or holding hands with a loved one. Accepting the transience of your life and its situations, and knowing that what you have in this moment is the most important thing, allows you to feel gratitude. Each night before you go to sleep think of at least two things from your day for which you are grateful. It is these moments of light within the darkness of your illness that can help to get you through each day.

Within the field of addictions, there is a common phrase used – take it one day at a time. When distressed, scale it back to 'take it one hour at a time' or 'take a minute at a time'. Tell yourself, 'I'll focus on the good, allow myself to laugh, be present with the person sitting with me, be happy, allow a sense of peace, be quiet inside' (or whatever it is you need).

Compassion and kindness

Coupled with gratitude is compassion, feeling and showing tenderness and softness towards suffering, particularly your suffering. You may feel uneasy showing kindness and compassion to yourself as you may not think you deserve it, or it's something that you give to others but not to yourself. You may feel ashamed about your condition and so don't believe you are worthy of compassion. Perhaps you need to learn how to give yourself this gentleness and care because without it, life can feel very harsh.

Being ill might mean that you can't do all that you would like to. It could mean less intimacy, fewer social interactions, not working, relying on others to manage financially and more. Without self-compassion there is too much room for self-criticism, judgement and self-hate. Compassion is the shoulder upon which you can lean so that you can reach your destination. Without it, getting through each day can seem like a battleground and when you are going through a difficult time, being compassionate and loving towards yourself will give you strength, endurance and nurturance.

Life without suffering

We suffer because we are human beings capable of it. Our suffering can help us to be understanding and empathetic towards others and what happens in their lives. However, when we attach so strongly to our expectations of life, people and outcomes, we run the risk of being disappointed and disgruntled. The 'if only' scenario plays through our minds and what we actually do have gets lost, forgotten about or pushed aside as insufficient. When we can manage our lives and separate them from the suffering that we attach to its experiences, we can begin to focus on all that we do have, even when it involves having cancer. Distress comes and goes, life comes and goes, but what remains constant is the realness of this moment for all that it brings. Be gentle and kind to yourself as each moment unfolds and passes.

You will notice that the more you do the practices, the greater the benefits. One of these benefits is that you can readily learn how to refocus your attention. Throughout the book and in the practices, there are several references to coming back, in a gentle and kind manner, to your anchor, to that part within you that is stable and balanced. When life is busy, when things get tough, when grief feels unbearable, when fear overwhelms you or you're feeling adrift, drop anchor. Make the association in your mind of that anchor always being there to ground you, to keep you steadfast and allowing for equanimity, for calm and balance in shifting times.

Live your life one breath at a time.

References

2 Cancer facts, figures and statistics

1 Cancer Research <www.cancerresearchuk.org/health-professional/
cancer-statistics-for-the-uk#heading-Three>

2 World Health Organization <www.who.int/cancer/en/>

3 Cancer Research UK <www.cancerresearchuk.org/health-professional/
cancer-statistics/worldwide-cancer#heading-Zero>

4 Cancer Research UK <www.cancerresearchuk.org/health-professional/
cancer-statistics/worldwide-cancer#heading-Zero>

5 Cancer Research UK <www.cancerresearchuk.org/health-professional/
cancer-statistics/worldwide-cancer#heading-Zero>

6 Cancer Research UK <www.cancerresearchuk.org/health-professional/
cancer-statistics/worldwide-cancer#heading-Zero>

7 National Cancer Institute <www.cancer.gov/about-cancer/treatment/types/>

8 Cancer Research UK <www.cancerresearchuk.org/health-professional/
cancer-statistics/survival/common-cancers-compared>

3 Mind and body

1 Nair, S., Sagar, M., Sollers, J., Consedine, N. and Broadbent, E. (2015), 'Do
slumped and upright postures affect stress responses? A randomized trial'.
Health Psychology 34(6), pp. 632–41.

2 Borrell-Carrió, F., Suchman, A. L. and Epstein, R. M. (2004), 'The Biopsychosocial Model 25 years later: principles, practice, and scientific inquiry'. *The
Annals of Family Medicine* 2(6), pp. 576–82.

3 Rezek, C. A. (2010), *Life Happens: Waking up to Yourself and Your Life in a
Mindful Way*, London: Leachcroft.

4 Mindfulness, meditation and cancer

1 Ott, M. J., Norris, R. L. and Bauer-Wu, S. M. (2006), 'Mindfulness meditation for oncology patients: a discussion and critical review'. *Integrative Cancer Therapies,* June 5(2), pp. 98–108.

2 Tacón, A. M., Caldera, Y. M. and Ronaghan, C. (2004), 'Mindfulness-Based Stress Reduction in women with breast cancer'. *Families, Systems, and Health* 22(2), pp. 193–203.

3 Ledesma, D. and Kumano, H. (2009), 'Mindfulness-based stress reduction and cancer: a meta-analysis'. *Psychooncology* 18(6).

4 Ledesma, D. and Kumano, H. (2009), 'Mindfulness-based stress reduction and cancer: a meta-analysis'. *Psychooncology* 18(6).

5 Matousek, R. H and Dobkin, P. L. (2010), 'Weathering storms: a cohort study of how participation in a Mindfulness-Based Stress Reduction program benefits women after breast cancer treatment'. *Current Oncology* 17(4), pp. 62–70.

6 Shennan, C., Payne S. and Fenlon, D. (2011), 'What is the evidence for the use of mindfulness-based interventions in cancer care? A review'. *Psychooncology* 20(7), pp. 681-97.

7 Chang, Y. Y., Wang, L. Y., Liu, C. Y., Chien, T. J., Chen, I. J. and Hsu, C. H. (2018), 'The effects of a mindfulness meditation program on quality of life in cancer outpatients: an exploratory study'. *Integrative Cancer Therapies* (17) 2.

8 Pollard, A., Burchell, J. L., Castle, D., Neilson, K., Ftanou, M., Corry, J., Rischin, D., Kissane, D. W., Krishnasamy, M., Carlson, L.E. and Couper, J. (2017), 'Individualised mindfulness-based stress reduction for head and neck cancer patients undergoing radiotherapy of curative intent: a descriptive pilot study'. *European Journal of Cancer Care* 26(2).

9 Johannsen, M., O'Connor, M., O'Toole, M. S., Jensen, A. B., Højris, I. and Zachariae, R. (2016), 'Efficacy of mindfulness-based cognitive therapy on late post-treatment pain in women treated for primary breast cancer: a randomized controlled trial'. *Journal of Clinical Oncology* 34(28).

10 Tacon, A. M. (2016), 'Brief mindfulness findings and cancer related pain'. *Journal of Alternative Medical Research* 2(2), p. 114.

11 Lengacher, C. A., Johnson-Mallard, V., Post-White, J., Moscoso, M. S., Jacobsen, P. B., Klein, T. W., Widen, R. H., Fitzgerald, S. G., Shelton, M. M., Barta, M., Goodman, M., Cox, C. E. and Kip, K. E. (2009), 'Randomized controlled trial of Mindfulness-Based Stress Reduction (MBSR) for survivors of breast cancer'. *Psychooncology* 18(12), pp. 1261–72.

12 Carlson, L.E., Ursuliak, Z., Goodey, E., Angen, M. and Speca, M. (2001), 'The effects of a mindfulness meditation-based stress reduction program on

mood and symptoms of stress in cancer outpatients 6-month follow up'. *Support Care Cancer* 9(2), pp. 112–23.

13 Speca, M., Carlson, L. E., Goodey, E. and Angen, M. (2000), 'A randomized, wait-list controlled clinical trial: the effect of a mindfulness meditation-based stress reduction program on mood and symptoms of stress in cancer outpatients'. *Psychosomatic Medicine* 62(5), pp. 613–22.

14 Lengacher, C. A., Johnson-Mallard, V., Post-White, J., Moscoso, M. S., Jacobsen, P. B., Klein, T. W., Widen, R. H., Fitzgerald, S. G., Shelton, M. M., Barta, M., Goodman, M., Cox, C. E. and Kip, K. E. (2009), 'Randomized controlled trial of Mindfulness-Based Stress Reduction (MBSR) for survivors of breast cancer'. *Psychooncology* 18(12), pp. 1261–72.

15 Reich, R. R., Lengacher, C. A., Alinat, C. B., Kip, K. E., Paterson, C., Ramesar, S., Han, H. S., Ismail-Khan, R., Johnson-Mallard, V., Moscoso, M., Budhrani-Shani, P., Shivers, S., Cox, C. E., Goodman, M. and Park, J. (2017), 'Mindfulness-Based Stress Reduction in post-treatment breast cancer patients: immediate and sustained effects across multiple symptom Clusters'. *Journal of Pain Symptom Management* 53(1), pp. 85–95.

16 Smith, J. E., Richardson, J., Hoffman, C. and Pilkington, K. (2005), 'Mindfulness-Based Stress Reduction as supportive therapy in cancer care: systematic review'. *Journal of Advanced Nursing* 52(3), pp. 315–27.

17 Sarenmalm, E. K., Mårtensson, L. B., Andersson, B. A., Karlsson, P. and Bergh, I. (2017), 'Mindfulness and its efficacy for psychological and biological responses in women with breast cancer'. *Cancer Medicine* 6(5), pp. 1108–22.

18 Cusens, B., Duggan, G. B., Thorne, K. et al. (2010), 'Evaluation of the Breathworks mindfulness-based pain management programme: effects on well-being and multiple measures of mindfulness'. *Clinical Psychology and Psychotherapy* 17(1), pp. 63–78.

19 Getting started with Metacognition, Cambridge Assessment, International Education <https://cambridge-community.org.uk/professional-development/gswmeta/index.html>

6 Fear, worry and anxiety

1 Yehuda, R., Resnick, H., Kahana, B. and Giller, E. L. (1993), 'Long-lasting hormonal alterations to extreme stress in humans: normative or maladaptive?' *Psychosomatic Medicine* 55(3), pp. 287–97.

2 Davidson, R. J., Jackson, D. C. and Kalin, N. H. (2000), 'Emotion, plasticity, context, and regulation: perspectives from affective neuroscience'. *Psychological Bulletin* 126(6), p. 890.

3 Stein, D. J. (2006), 'Advances in understanding the anxiety disorders: the cognitive-affective neuroscience of "false alarms"'. *Annals of Clinical Psychiatry: Official Journal of the American Academy of Clinical Psychiatrists* 18(3), p. 173.

4 Pyszczynski, T., Hamilton, J. C., Herring, F. H. and Greenberg, J. (1989), 'Depression, self-focused attention, and the negative memory bias'. *Journal of Personality and Social Psychology* 57(2), pp. 351–7.

5 Clarke, P., MacLeod, C. and Shirazee, N. (2008), 'Prepared for the worst: readiness to acquire threat bias and susceptibility to elevate trait anxiety'. *Emotion* 8(1), p. 47.

6 Joormann, J., Dkane, M. and Gotlib, I. H. (2006), 'Adaptive and maladaptive components of rumination? Diagnostic specificity and relation to depressive biases'. *Behavior Therapy* 37(3), pp. 269–80.

7 Stress

1 Hölzel, B. K., Carmody, J., Vangel, M., Congleton, C., Yerramsetti, S. M., Gard, T. and Lazar, S. W. (2011), 'Mindfulness practice leads to increases in regional brain gray matter density'. *Psychiatry Research: Neuroimaging* 191(1), pp. 36–43.

2 Coffey, K. A., Hartman, M. and Fredrickson, B. L. (2010), 'Deconstructing mindfulness and constructing mental health: understanding mindfulness and its mechanisms of action'. *Mindfulness* 1(4), pp. 235–53.

3 Pressley, M., Wood, E., Woloshyn, V. E., Martin, V., King, A. and Menke, D. (1992), 'Encouraging mindful use of prior knowledge: attempting to construct explanatory answers facilitates learning'. *Educational Psychologist* 27(1), pp. 91–109.

4 Heeren, A., Van Broeck, N. and Philippot, P. (2009), 'The effects of mindfulness on executive processes and autobiographical memory specificity'. *Behaviour Research and Therapy* 47(5), pp. 403–9.

5 Brown, K. W. and Ryan, R. M. (2003), 'The benefits of being present: mindfulness and its role in psychological well-being'. *Journal of Personality and Social Psychology* 84(4), p. 822.

6 Academic Mindfulness Interest Group. (2006), 'Mindfulness-based psychotherapies: a review of conceptual foundations, empirical evidence and practical considerations'. *Australian and New Zealand Journal of Psychiatry* 40(4), pp. 285–94.

7 Davidson, R. J., Kabat-Zinn, J., Schumacher, J., Rosenkranz, M., Muller, D., Santorelli, S. F. and Sheridan, J. F. (2003), 'Alterations in brain and immune function produced by mindfulness meditation'. *Psychosomatic Medicine* 65(4), pp. 564–70.

8 Shapiro, S. L., Carlson, L. E., Astin, J. A. and Freedman, B. (2006), 'Mechanisms of mindfulness'. *Journal of Clinical Psychology* 62(3), pp. 373–86.

11 Self-care

1 Robinson, L., Smith, M. and Segal, J. 'Laughter is the best medicine'. <www.helpguide.org/articles/mental-health/laughter-is-the-best-medicine.htm>

12 Memories, pain, sleep and exercise

1 Rezek, C. A. (2016), *Pain Management: The Mindful Way*. London: Sheldon Press.

2 Wiesenfeld-Hallin, Z. (2005), 'Sex differences in pain perception'. *Gender Medicine* 2(3), pp. 137–45.

3 Rezek, C. (2011), 'The different angles of pain'. *Pain News*, pp. 29–31. <www.lifehappens-mindfulness.com/wp-content/uploads/2013/02/The-Different-Angles-of-Pain-enc_painarticle.pdf>

4 Zeidan, F., Emerson, N., Farris, S., Ray, J., Jung, Y., McHaffie, J. and Coghill, R. (2015), 'Mindfulness meditation-based pain relief employs different neural mechanisms than placebo and sham mindfulness meditation-induced analgesia'. *Journal of Neuroscience* 5(46), pp. 15307–25.

5 Cherkin, D. C., Sherman, K. J., Balderson, B. H et al. (2016), 'Effect of mindfulness-based stress reduction vs cognitive behavioral therapy or usual care on back pain and functional limitations in adults with chronic low back pain: a randomized clinical trial'. *Journal of the American Medical Association* 315(12), pp. 1240–9.

6 Melzack, R and Wall, P. D. (1965), 'Pain mechanisms: a new theory'. *Science* 150(3699), pp. 971–9.

7 Derbyshire NHS Trust, Health Psychology Service. (2012), The Gate Control Theory.

8 Moore, S. C., Lee, I. M., Weiderpass, E., Campbell, P. T., Sampson, J. N., Kitahara, C. M., Keadle, S. K., Arem, H., Berrington de Gonzalez, A., Hartge, P., Adami, H. O., Blair, C. K., Borch, K. B., Boyd, E., Check, D. P., Fournier, A., Freedman, N. D., Gunter, M., Johannson, M., Khaw, K. T., Linet, M. S., Orsini, N., Park, Y., Riboli, E., Robien, K., Schairer, C., Sesso, H., Spriggs, M., Van Dusen, R., Wolk, A., Matthews, C. E. and Patel, A. V. (2016), 'Leisure-time physical activity and risk of 26 types of cancer in 1.44 million adults'. *JAMA Internal Medicine* 176(6), pp. 816–25.

9 Bernstein, L., Patel, A. V., Ursin, G., Sullivan-Halley, J., Press, M. F., Deapen, D., Berlin, J. A., Daling, J. R., McDonald, J. A., Norman, S. A., Malone,

K. E., Strom, B. L., Liff, J., Folger, S. G., Simon, M. S., Burkman, R. T., Marchbanks, P. A., Weiss, L. K. and Spirtas, R. (2015), 'Lifetime recreational exercise activity and breast cancer risk among black women and white women'. *Journal of the National Cancer Institute* 97(22), pp. 1671–9.

10 Wolin, K.Y., Yan, Y. and Colditz, G. A. (2011), 'Physical activity and risk of colon adenoma: a meta-analysis'. *British Journal of Cancer* 104(5), pp. 882–5.

11 Yang, Z., Gottlieb, L., Cartmel, B., Li, F., Ercolano, E. A., Harrigan, M., McCorkle, R., Ligibel, J. A., Von Gruenigen, V. E., Gogoi, R., Schwartz, P. E., Risch, H. A., Irwin, M. L. (2017), 'Randomized trial of exercise on quality of life in women with ovarian cancer: women's activity and lifestyle study in Connecticut (WALC)'. *Journal of the National Cancer Institute* 109(12).

12 Courneya, K. S., McKenzie, D. C., Mackey, J. R., Gelmon, K., Friedenreich, C. M., Yasui, Y., Reid, R. D., Cook, D., Jespersen, D., Proulx, C., Dolan, L. B., Forbes, C. C., Wooding, E., Trinh, L. and Segal, R. J. (2013), 'Effects of exercise dose and type during breast cancer chemotherapy: multicenter randomized trial'. *Journal of the National Cancer Institute* 105(23), pp 1821–32.

13 Vainio, H., Kaaks, R. and Bianchini, F. (2002), 'Weight control and physical activity in cancer prevention: international evaluation of the evidence'. *European Journal of Cancer Prevention* 11(2), pp. S94–100.

14 Moore, S. C., Gierach, G. L., Schatzkin, A. and Matthews, C. E. (2010), 'Physical activity, sedentary behaviours, and the prevention of endometrial cancer'. *British Journal of Cancer* 103(7), pp. 933–8.

15 Steindorf, K., Ritte, R., Eomois, P. P., Lukanova, A., Tjonneland, A., Johnsen, N. F., Overvad, K., Østergaard, J. N., Clavel-Chapelon, F., Fournier, A., Dossus, L., Teucher, B., Rohrmann, S., Boeing, H., Wientzek, A., Trichopoulou, A., Karapetyan, T., Trichopoulos, D., Masala, G., Berrino, F., Mattiello, A., Tumino, R., Ricceri, F., Quirós, J. R., Travier, N., Sánchez, M. J., Navarro, C., Ardanaz, E., Amiano, P., Bueno-de-Mesquita, H. B., van Duijnhoven, F., Monninkhof, E., May, A. M., Khaw, K. T., Wareham, N., Key, T. J., Travis, R. C., Borch, K. B., Sund, M., Andersson, A., Fedirko, V., Rinaldi, S., Romieu, I., Wahrendorf, J., Riboli, E. and Kaaks, R. (2013), 'Physical activity and risk of breast cancer overall and by hormone receptor status: the European prospective investigation into cancer and nutrition'. *International Journal of Cancer Care* 132(7), pp. 1667–78.

16 Fournier, A., Dos Santos, G., Guillas, G., Bertsch, J., Duclos, M., Boutron-Ruault, M. C., Clavel-Chapelon, F. and Mesrine, S. (2014), 'Recent recreational physical activity and breast cancer risk in postmenopausal women in the E3N cohort'. *Cancer Epidemiology, Biomarkers and Prevention:*

A Publication of the American Association for Cancer Research 23(9), pp. 1893–902.

17 Wu, Y., Zhang, D. and Kang, S. (2013), 'Physical activity and risk of breast cancer: a meta-analysis of prospective studies'. *Breast Cancer Research Treatment* 137(3), pp. 869–82.

18 Liu, Y., Hu, F., Li, D., Wang, F., Zhu, L., Chen, W., Ge, J., An, R. and Zhao, Y. (2011), 'Does physical activity reduce the risk of prostate cancer? A systematic review and meta-analysis'. *European Urology* 60(5), pp. 1029–44.

19 Buffart, L. M., Singh, A. S., van Loon, E. C., Vermeulen, H. I., Brug, J. and Chinapaw, M.J. (2014), 'Physical activity and the risk of developing lung cancer among smokers: a meta-analysis'. *Journal of Science and Medicine in Sport* 17(1), pp. 67–71.

20 Friedenreich, C. M., Neilson, H. K. and Lynch, B. M. (2010), 'State of the epidemiological evidence on physical activity and cancer prevention'. *European Journal of Cancer* 46(14), pp. 2593–604.

21 Burnham, T. R. and Wilcox, A. (2002), 'Effects of exercise on physiological and psychological variables in cancer survivors'. *Medicine and Science in Sports and Exercise* 34(12), pp. 1863–1867.

13 Get moving

1 University College London, School of Pharmacy (2012), *Relieving Persistent Pain: Improving Health Outcomes*. London: UCL.

14 Gratitude

1 Emmons, R. A. and McCullough, M. E. (2003), 'Counting blessings versus burdens: an experimental investigation of gratitude and subjective well-being in daily life'. *Journal of Personality and Social Psychology* 84(2), pp. 377–389.

2 Froh, J. J., Sefick, W. J. and Emmons, R. A. (2008), 'Counting blessings in early adolescents: an experimental study of gratitude and subjective well-being'. *Journal of School Psychology* 46(2), pp. 213–33.

3 Ng, M. and Wong, W. (2013), 'The differential effects of gratitude and sleep on psychological distress in patients with chronic pain'. *Journal of Health Psychology* 18(2), pp. 263–71.

4 Wood, A. M., Froh, J. J. and Geraghty, A. W. (2010), 'Gratitude and well-being: a review and theoretical integration'. *Clinical Psychology Review* 30(7), pp. 890–905.

1637665

QUEEN MARGARET COLLEGE

LIBRARY

Please return book on or before latest date
stamped below